# DASH DIET *for*
# RENAL
# HEALTH

T0109053

# DASH DIET *for* RENAL HEALTH

A Customized Program
to Improve Your
Kidney Function
Based on America's
Top-Rated Diet

**Sara Monk Rivera, RD**
**Kristin Diversi, MS**

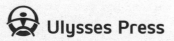 Ulysses Press

Published in the United States by:
ULYSSES PRESS
P.O. Box 3440
Berkeley, CA 94703
www.ulyssespress.com

ISBN: 978-1-61243-784-2
Library of Congress Control Number: 2018930784

Printed in Canada by Marquis Book Printing
10 9 8 7 6 5 4 3 2 1

Acquisitions editor: Bridget Thoreson
Managing editor: Claire Chun
Editor: Renee Rutledge
Proofreader: Shayna Keyles
Indexer: Sayre van Young
Production: Jake Flaherty
Front cover design: Rebecca Lown
Cover artwork: hummus and vegetables © JeniFoto/shutterstock.com, salmon © Timolina/
    shutterstock.com; fruits and vegetables © Serg64/shutterstock.com
Interior artwork: kidney page 10 © Sakurra/shutterstock.com, hands page 83
    Lyudmyla Kharlamova/shutterstock.com

Distributed by Publishers Group West

NOTE TO READERS: This book has been written and published strictly for informational and educational purposes only. It is not intended to serve as medical advice or to be any form of medical treatment. You should always consult your physician before altering or changing any aspect of your medical treatment and/or undertaking a diet regimen, including the guidelines as described in this book. Do not stop or change any prescription medications without the guidance and advice of your physician. Any use of the information in this book is made on the reader's good judgment after consulting with his or her physician and is the reader's sole responsibility. This book is not intended to diagnose or treat any medical condition and is not a substitute for a physician.

This book is independently authored and published and no sponsorship or endorsement of this book by, and no affiliation with, any trademarked brands or other products mentioned within is claimed or suggested. All trademarks that appear in ingredient lists and elsewhere in this book belong to their respective owners and are used here for informational purposes only. The authors and publisher encourage readers to patronize the quality brands mentioned and pictured in this book.

# CONTENTS

# INTRODUCTION

When you have kidney issues or your kidney health is compromised, you need to have a nutrition plan that accommodates your needs. But that doesn't mean depriving yourself or giving up the things you love. You just need to learn how to make simple adjustments in your diet to enjoy better kidney function.

When you were first diagnosed with kidney disease, you may not have been told to reduce fluids (anything that is liquid at room temperature) and certain nutrients, such as sodium, phosphorous, potassium, or protein. However, if your kidney disease state has worsened, you will need to pay careful attention to the foods you consume, and may be told by your doctor or dietitian to reduce your intake of certain nutrients. This is called a renal diet.

Your kidneys are responsible for filtering bodily fluids, excreting waste, and much more. When your kidneys aren't functioning properly, waste and fluid from food and liquids you consume can build up in your body. This is why certain nutrients must be limited—to reduce the amount of waste in your blood. In simpler terms, processing certain nutrients can become too difficult for your body, which can lead to toxicity if you don't follow your prescribed diet properly.

A renal diet can be intimidating at first. However, it is crucial to follow your individual dietary advice because waste and fluid built up in your body can cause other health problems, especially for your heart and bones.

The guidelines and recommendations within this book are founded on scientific evidence that prove the DASH (Dietary Approaches to Stop Hypertension) diet, although originally designed to lower blood pressure, is also effective for lowering cholesterol, managing or preventing diabetes, reducing the risk of kidney stone formation, aiding in weight loss, and lowering the risk for additional diseases such as heart disease, stroke, and cancer.

The DASH diet, recommended by the National Kidney Foundation, is an eating plan that encourages the consumption of a variety of real, whole foods daily—and that's why we love it. As nutritionists, our goal for this book is to break down the science of the diet in a basic and approachable manner so you can understand why it has been ranked the best diet for the seventh year in a row by the *U.S. News and World Report*. Thirty-eight diets were considered, and in order to receive high ratings, a diet had to be simple to follow, healthy, safe, and an efficient way to lose weight and guard against conditions such as type 2 diabetes and heart disease.

This book will provide vital information on how to successfully follow the DASH diet to improve renal, or kidney, health issues. However, the DASH diet isn't really a diet—it's a lifestyle. If you're willing to implement the recommendations in this book, you will see results and improve your overall health. It takes time to break habits and to get accustomed to new foods, but if you are willing to do it slowly and correctly, you will change your entire lifestyle for the better. Small steps will lead you to sustainable lifestyle changes. Even if you make one good behavior or dietary change per week, you'll be on the right path.

By learning how to successfully follow the DASH diet, you'll help much more than your kidneys. You'll help your blood pressure, heart health, and body mass index (BMI). Basically, you'll be working to improve your overall health—and that's something we should all be aiming to do!

In this book, we're going to:
- Provide easy, go-to lists of specific foods that you should avoid or limit when you have kidney issues. This will come in handy,

especially when food shopping or choosing what to eat at a restaurant.

- Offer safe substitutions and recommendations that you can include in your meal planning and meals out so you can enjoy eating without feeling restricted or deprived.

- Explain *how* and *why* these changes to your diet will help improve your kidney health and the quality of your life.

This book will help you implement the DASH diet in an adaptable and flexible manner to fit your nutritional needs and desires. We're going to provide you with meal options and tools to successfully get meals on the table without frustration, and more importantly, without getting bored. You'll get lists of breakfasts, lunches, dinners, and snacks. We'll provide you with tips, such as how to eat mindfully, use spices and herbs instead of salt to flavor food, and make healthy swaps to the meals you love. In addition, you'll get shopping lists broken down by food group, as well as shopping tips, such as keeping to the perimeter of the supermarket to avoid purchasing processed, prepackaged foods in the middle aisles.

Whether you're the type of person to plan your meals for the upcoming month or wing it day by day, you'll have DASH diet meals laid out for you so you can pick and choose your menu items. By the end of this book, you'll be a bit more organized, understand how to plan ahead, and enjoy the process of purchasing and preparing your own meals.

Changing your eating habits isn't always simple or desirable, but it's almost always necessary. Our food supply, food systems, and the unlimited access we have to processed, high-sodium, high-sugar foods can make it very difficult to comply with a healthy eating regimen. However, you're here, reading this book, bettering yourself and your health. You have already taken the first step, the hardest step, which is why we know you are motivated enough to do this. Even if you are reading this book to learn more about a friend or family member's kidney condition, you can benefit from this book. The DASH diet is not just for those with hypertension or kidney issues; it is for everybody and anybody. We can all benefit from consuming real, whole foods and adopting an overall healthy eating plan.

From this point on, you can stop feeling bad about your eating habits and learn how to slowly change them until it becomes a lifestyle. We'll discuss not only why falling off track a few times is okay, but also how to learn from it. Creating a new lifestyle for yourself will not happen overnight; it's a learning process that will take time, but the healthy habits you develop will allow you to be the healthiest version of yourself and prevent health issues down the road. There is nothing more important than your individual health.

*Chapter 1*

# THE IMPORTANCE OF KIDNEY HEALTH

Your kidneys are two bean-shaped organs located just below your rib cage, with one on either side of your spine (think: the middle of your lower back area). Directly on top of each kidney are the adrenal glands, small glands that produce hormones (chemicals released into the blood to trigger or regulate a particular function of the body), such as sex hormones and cortisol. Cortisol helps you respond to stress and has many other important functions.

## What Kidneys Do

The kidneys filter about 120 to 150 quarts of blood to produce 1 to 2 quarts of urine daily. Picture your kidneys as your body's internal filtration system.

Good kidney function is essential for maintaining homeostasis in your body. Homeostasis can be defined as the tendency of an organism or cell to regulate its internal conditions to stabilize health and functioning. So, as changes occur, the body works hard to maintain uniform conditions, such as body temperature, blood pH, and the amount of glucose in the blood.

Your kidneys are specifically responsible for maintaining proper pH levels and electrolyte balance. Electrolytes are minerals that carry an electric charge when dissolved in a liquid, such as blood. Sodium, potassium, chloride, and bicarbonate are the blood electrolytes that help regulate nerve and muscle function. They also maintain acid-base balance and water balance, which will be discussed shortly.

Cells are life's basic unit of structure and function. A balance between fluids and electrolytes is necessary for cells to function properly and survive. The amount of electrolytes in the body influences the amount of fluid because when electrolyte levels are high, the body retains more water, which in turn increases the volume of blood. Picture this: Water follows sodium. This causes an increase in the amount of water in the body and volume of blood in circulation. More blood volume results in blood pressure climbing up. Excess sodium, and in turn, excess water, prevents blood vessels from easily contracting and relaxing. When the body loses water, the kidneys will conserve it by only producing a small amount of concentrated urine (you know, the kind that usually smells and is dark yellow).

On the other hand, when one consumes excess water, the kidneys produce large amounts of urine to maintain the electrolyte balance and rid the body of excess water. In other words, when one consumes excess water, the kidneys produce large amounts of urine to maintain the balance.

The kidneys also produce hormone-like substances called prostaglandins, which are made from lipid, commonly known as fat. These substances aid in the stimulation of the production of renin. Renin is an enzyme produced by the kidneys that plays an important role in the renin-angiotensin-aldosterone hormonal system responsible for controlling blood pressure. It's a bit complicated, but we'll break it down as simply as possible.

## Renin-Angiotensin-Aldosterone System

The body has many systems that work together to maintain homeostasis, and this system is one of them. It has three functions:

1. To maintain proper blood pressure/blood flow
2. To maintain the right concentration of sodium in the blood
3. To maintain the right amount of water in the blood

The start of the system occurs when the juxtaglomerular apparatus, which are cells located next to the glomerulus in the kidney, sense low blood pressure and blood flow. Decreased blood flow can be caused by sodium or water loss (from diarrhea, vomiting, or excessive perspiration) or by a narrowing of a renal artery.

A decrease in sodium reduces the amount of water in the blood, meaning the blood pressure is lowered. In response to this, the glomerulus releases renin into the bloodstream. Renin moves to the liver and starts the conversion of angiotensinogen, an inactive protein, into active angiotensin I. Angiotensin I then travels to the lungs where an enzyme called angiotensin converting enzyme (ACE) converts angiotensin I into angiotensin II.

Angiotensin II has the ability to constrict blood vessels, which in turn increases blood pressure. The other function of angiotensin II is to stimulate the secretion of aldosterone, a steroid hormone secreted by the adrenal glands. Remember, the adrenal glands are glands on top of the kidneys.

Aldosterone, the regulator of salt and water balance in the body, then stimulates sodium reabsorption by the kidneys. Reabsorption means the substances are being absorbed again; thus, they are returning and being used by the kidneys once more.

When aldosterone increases sodium reabsorption, water and chloride follow, and blood volume is increased. Chloride is crucial to this process because it's needed to maintain proper acid-base balance. Also, just like sodium, chloride is an extracellular electrolyte. Sodium and chloride work together to control extracellular volume and blood pressure. Increased blood volume can trigger the release of a hormone called atrial natriuretic hormone (ANH), which inhibits the release of aldosterone. This keeps the body's water and sodium levels at the homeostatic levels. Overall, this pathway shows that water follows highly concentrated electrolytes. Ultimately, the kidneys work hard to balance water and solutes and control blood pressure.

# Your Kidney Is Like a Water Filter

Your kidneys are responsible for filtering blood and flushing waste products through urine. This is why it's important to drink adequate water daily. Water helps to keep things moving, flowing, and flushing. In fact, chronic low-grade dehydration is one of the most common causes of kidney stones.

Symptoms of dehydration include:

- Thirst
- Dry skin
- Fatigue and weakness
- Increased body temperature
- Muscle cramping
- Headaches
- Nausea
- Dark-colored urine
- Dry mouth, nose, or eyes

Severe dehydration may also include:

- Muscle spasms
- Vomiting
- Vision issues
- Loss of consciousness
- Kidney or liver failure

Dehydration compromises cellular efficiency and, ultimately, your health. It is common in many patients we see. This is partially due to the fact that our patients count their cups of tea and coffee toward their water intake. But coffee and tea actually have a mild diuretic effect on the body, meaning they cause your body to release more urine. Although they are not strong contributors to dehydration, they should never replace plain, clean water. When you are thirsty, drink water. Nothing else. And, hopefully, you won't get to the point of being thirsty. A good, general daily goal for water intake should be eight to ten 8-ounce glasses, as long as you're not on a fluid restriction.

When the kidneys don't function properly, waste products and excess fluid can build up. Also, sodium, potassium, phosphorous, and calcium aren't regulated correctly. The buildup of these substances may cause the symptoms of kidney disease, including:

- High blood pressure
- Excessive tiredness (lethargy)
- Fluid retention
- Lower back pain

Ultimately, kidney damage can be a result of diabetes, high blood pressure, and infections. Other dietary factors, such as excessive protein intake, are believed to threaten kidney health. You may have seen people chugging down their protein shakes or chomping down on their protein bars, even after including steak, chicken, and eggs in all of their meals. The truth is, your body does not need that excess protein. Excessive protein intake is concerning for individuals with preexisting renal disease; however, studies have not proven a link between protein intake and the initiation or progression of renal disease in healthy individuals. So, while excess protein is not necessary, studies do not show that it initiates kidney disease. Evidence does show that changes in renal function from protein is likely a normal adaptive mechanism. While there is no sufficient evidence to restrict dietary protein intake in healthy individuals for the sake of preserving kidney function, it is not warranted to consume excess amounts either. In other words, include protein in your meals, but don't use supplemental protein shakes and drinks. And, quite frankly, they're usually a waste of money!

Waste products, which are materials your body can't use or has already broken down, such as protein, are removed and eliminated by the kidneys through urine. Urine includes multiple components, such as urea and uric acid (a byproduct of protein and fructose), which are produced from the breakdown of proteins. Both protein and fructose can increase these byproducts (fructose is the scientific name for honey or fruit sugar). It is common for people to consume excess protein and fructose. Most Americans consume three to five times more protein than needed and two to four times more fructose.[1]

Evidently, the kidney has many roles in the body, which is why kidney health is so very important. As you now know, poor kidney function is associated with other chronic health issues, including diabetes, hypertension, and heart disease. This means that eating a healthful, balanced diet can preserve kidney function and delay other medical issues.

---

1  Joseph Mercola, "How to Prevent and Treat Kidney Health with Food," Mercola.com, February 15, 2016, http://articles.mercola.com/sites/articles/archive/2016/02/15/foods-for-kidney-health.aspx.

# Healthy Kidneys Versus Unhealthy Kidneys

It's important to understand the anatomy and physiology of kidneys. The more you understand how your body functions, the more you'll understand the importance of the health of your organs, bones, muscles, and more, and the more likely you'll mindfully fuel your body with the proper foods to make it run efficiently.

The kidneys contain nephrons, which are millions of microscopic filters. This is why we refer to your kidneys as a water filter. Picture nephrons as a colander (the kitchen item you put pasta in after boiling to strain the liquid out). Nephrons allow fluid and waste products to pass through, but hold on to blood cells and large molecules to be returned to the bloodstream. The fluid and waste that pass through are removed as urine.

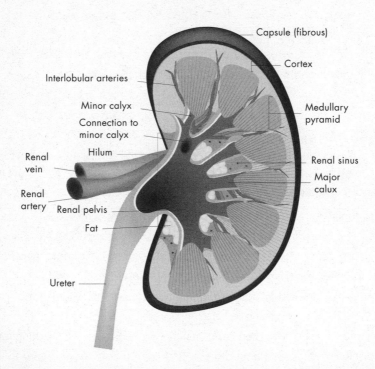

Interlobular arteries

Minor calyx

Connection to minor calyx

Hilum

Renal vein

Renal artery

Renal pelvis

Fat

Ureter

Capsule (fibrous)

Cortex

Medullary pyramid

Renal sinus

Major calux

# Tests to Indicate Kidney Health

Several tests and measurements, including lab work and urine samples, can indicate how your kidneys are functioning. It's important to be aware of the desirable ranges for each test.

**Glomerular Filtration Rate.** Chronic kidney disease (CKD) is a permanent, progressive loss of kidney function characterized by a decline in total glomerular filtration rate (GFR). Testing the GFR is crucial, as it indicates how well the kidneys are filtering and how well the nephrons are operating. It's particularly important to know your GFR if you are at risk for kidney disease.

The National Kidney Foundation Kidney Disease Outcome Quality Initiative classifies CKD into five stages based on GFR level. The GFR is measured by milliliters per minute (m/L/min). If and when stage 5 is reached, dialysis is needed.

## STAGES OF CHRONIC KIDNEY DISEASE

| Stage of CKD | GFR (m/L/min) |
| --- | --- |
| 1 | >90 |
| 2 | 60–89 |
| 3 | 30–59 |
| 3A | 45–59 |
| 3B | 30–44 |
| 4 | 15–29 |
| 5 | <15 |

In stage 1 of CKD, GFR is 90 or above, which is normal. However, abnormal levels of protein are detected in the urine.

In stage 5, the last stage of kidney disease, or end stage renal disease (ESRD), the kidneys have little function left.

Although stage 4 indicates a severe decrease in kidney function, you're still able to live without dialysis. While you cannot raise your GFR, you can prevent it from going lower. Because there's no cure for kidney disease, the primary focus is to stay nourished and reduce waste from building up.

**Serum Creatinine.** Creatinine is a waste product in your blood that comes from the metabolism of muscle cells. Healthy kidneys remove it from your blood and bring it into the urine to be excreted. With kidney dysfunction, the creatinine level rises as it builds up in the blood when kidneys aren't properly filtering blood (as you now know, this is shown with GFR test). Your health care provider can use the results of this test to calculate your GFR if your blood test results do not include it. A healthy level is below 1.2 milligrams per deciliter for women and 1.4 milligrams per deciliter for men. Higher levels can be an indication that the kidneys are not functioning properly.

**Creatinine Clearance.** This test measures how much creatinine is in your urine. It provides an accurate measurement of your kidneys' ability to remove creatinine from your body. You may be asked to save your urine for 24 hours and bring it to the lab. The normal value is greater than 90 milliliters per minute (mL/min). Milliliter per minute measures the rate at which one milliliter of matter crosses a surface during the time period equal to one minute.

**Blood Urea Nitrogen (BUN).** Blood carries protein to cells throughout the body. When the cells are done using the protein, the waste product returns to the blood and is named urea nitrogen. As with creatinine, urea nitrogen is normally removed from the blood and is excreted as urine by your kidneys. As the pattern goes, when there is kidney dysfunction, blood urea nitrogen (BUN) levels rise as it stays in your blood.

Normal BUN levels are 7 to 20 milligrams per deciliter (mg/dL). Levels greater than 20 mg/dL may indicate your kidneys are not functioning properly. Note that BUN may also rise if you consume excess protein in the diet; conversely, it can be low if you have inadequate protein intake. Elevated BUN may also be due to dehydration and heart failure.

**Urine Protein.** With kidney dysfunction, protein leaks into your urine. This condition is called proteinuria. This test should always be negative. Persistent protein in the urine is an early sign of CKD.

**Microalbumin Urine.** This is another test that can detect a very small amount of protein in your urine. With healthy kidneys, waste is removed from the blood but protein remains. Impaired kidneys may not separate a blood protein, called albumin, from the waste, so it removes it by excreting it in urine. In the beginning, only a very small amount of protein (which cannot be measured with a standard dipstick) may leak into the urine. This condition is called microalbuminuria, otherwise known as microalbumin in the urine.

Less than 30 mg/L is normal, greater than 30 mg/L but less than 300 mg/L is microalbuminuria, and greater than 300 mg/L is macroalbuminuria.

**Serum Albumin.** Albumin is the most common protein found in the blood, created from the protein you consume in your diet. It provides the body with the protein necessary to maintain growth and repair tissues. A low level of albumin indicates inadequate protein intake or overall inadequate calorie intake. A low serum albumin level can lead to health problems, such as inability to fight infections.

# Chronic Kidney Disease (CKD)

CKD means your kidneys are damaged and cannot filter blood properly. Chronic means that the damage to your kidneys happens slowly over a long period of time. This is the opposite of the term acute, which means the condition is severe and has a sudden onset. With CKD, your kidneys are unable to appropriately filter extra water and waste out of your blood to make urine, and waste builds up in the body. This can lead to other health issues. Diabetes and high blood pressure are the most common risk factors of kidney disease. Your health care provider will do tests to find out why you developed kidney disease, as the cause may influence the treatment you receive. Stay on top of getting annual bloodwork because the sooner you know about a disease, the sooner you can get treatment.

Following diabetes and high blood pressure, glomerulonephritis is the third most common type of kidney disease. It's a group of diseases that cause inflammation and damage to the kidney's filtering units (the glomeruli). Also, systemic lupus and other diseases that affect the body's immune system can cause CKD. Lupus is a chronic inflammatory disease that occurs when your body's own immune system attacks your tissues and organs. Congenital (a disease present from birth) malformations, obstructions due to kidney stones, tumors, an enlarged prostate gland in men, genetic diseases such as polycystic kidney, or frequent urinary tract infections are also causes of CKD.

It's crucial for those with CKD to be under the care of their health care provider and dietitian. Issues that may develop are the following:

- Protein-energy undernutrition, previously called protein-energy malnutrition. This is an energy deficit due to deficiency of all macronutrients (protein, fat, or carbs) and, many times, micronutrients as well. Micronutrients (vitamins and minerals) are needed in small amounts but are crucial for metabolism, heartbeat, bone density, and more.

- Changes in the metabolism of certain nutrients such as calcium, phosphorous, and vitamin D.

- Electrolyte and fluid imbalances, which are associated with hypertension, edema, congestive heart failure, and hyperkalemia (very high potassium, which is life threatening).

- Dyslipidemia and abnormal carbohydrate metabolism.

- Inability for the kidneys to produce erythropoietin, which can cause low iron stores and, ultimately, anemia.

## Diabetes and CKD

Now that you understand why high blood pressure can lead to kidney disease, let's review why diabetes can lead to it. Diabetes is a disease in which your body does not make enough insulin or cannot use normal amounts of insulin properly. Insulin is a hormone that regulates the amount of sugar in the blood.

There are two types of diabetes, type 1 and type 2. Twenty to 30% of patients with type 1 and type 2 diabetes have diabetic nephropathy, or diabetes-induced kidney disease.[2]

Type 1 diabetes often occurs in children, which is why another name for it is juvenile-onset diabetes mellitus. Because the pancreas does not make enough insulin and insulin injections are required, it is also named insulin-dependent diabetes.

Type 2 diabetes is the most common type. According to the CDC, an estimated 30.3 million people of all ages (9.4% of the US population) had diabetes in 2015.[3] Unlike with type 1 diabetes, for these cases, the pancreas does make insulin but it is used improperly by the body. Most times, high blood sugar levels can be controlled with a balanced diet, but many people choose to take medicine and insulin.

With diabetes, small blood vessels throughout the body are injured. Injured blood vessels in the kidney cannot clean blood properly, and waste materials build up in the blood. Diabetes can also damage the nerves in the body. This can cause difficulty emptying the bladder, and the pressure can injure the kidneys. Also, when urine remains in the bladder, infections can develop from bacteria thriving in the high-sugar environment.

One of the earliest signs of diabetic kidney disease is an increased excretion of albumin in the urine. This test is important to get done yearly because albumin is present long before other tests indicate kidney disease. Other signs include weight gain, ankle swelling, frequent urination, and high blood pressure. Blood, urine, and blood pressure should be checked at least once a year to treat high blood pressure and kidney disease early.

2   Heshmatollah Shahbazian and Isa Rezaii, "Diabetic Kidney Disease; Review of the Current Knowledge," *Journal of Renal Injury Prevention* 2, no. 2 (2013): 73[en]80, doi: 10.12861/jrip.2013.24.
3   Centers for Disease Control and Prevention, National Diabetes Statistics Report, 2017, Atlanta, GA: Centers for Disease Control and Prevention, US Department of Health and Human Services; 2017, https://www.cdc.gov/diabetes/pdfs/data/statistics/national-diabetes-statistics-report.pdf.

# How Does CKD Affect Your Everyday Life?

If you've learned you have kidney disease, you may feel you are doomed to dialysis and a boatload of weekly doctor visits. This isn't true. While kidney disease is progressive, meaning it can get worse over time, you have the power to prevent further damage and protect your kidneys by modifying your diet, including tons of nutritious and kidney-friendly foods, and adding healthy habits to your daily routine. You can still live a productive life and be physically active! The amazing thing about the body is that it responds well when we treat it well and fuel it properly.

*Chapter 2*

# OVERVIEW OF THE DASH DIET

The DASH diet was founded when researchers were testing nutrients as they occur together in food, and how they affected blood pressure. Called "DASH," an acronym for Dietary Approaches to Stop Hypertension, the study showed that blood pressure was reduced with a diet that emphasized fruits, vegetables, whole grains, fish, poultry, low-fat dairy products, beans, seeds, and nuts. It called for a reduction in the intake of red meat, high-fat foods, sweets, and sugary beverages. This research, however, was solely focused on stopping hypertension, and was not designed for weight loss, so it was high in refined grains and starchy foods. This is because the research was based on ideologies of nutrition in the 1990s, which is known in the nutrition world as the "low-fat era" (we'll discuss low-fat food products on page 48). Fortunately, new DASH diet research has been conducted.

One of the first DASH studies experimented with the effect of reduced dietary sodium intake on blood pressure. It involved 412 participants who were randomly assigned one of two eating plans: the DASH eating plan or the standard American diet (SAD). They followed the diet plans for a month for each of three sodium levels. The daily sodium levels in milligrams (mg) were the following: 3,300 milligrams per day (average amount of sodium consumed for most Americans), 2,300 milligrams, and 1,500 milligrams. For both eating plans, blood pressure was lowered with reduced sodium intake. At each sodium level, blood pressure was lower on the DASH diet that on the SAD. This means that although the sodium levels were the same, the body, most specifically the kidneys, responded well to the combination of nutrients from the DASH foods. Furthermore, the greatest blood pressure reduction overall was from the DASH diet at the sodium level of 1,500 milligrams.[4] This is why if you have hypertension, it is recommended to consume 1,500 milligrams of sodium per day.

It's wise of you to read a newly published book on the DASH diet and kidney health, as we are writing with the most current science-backed evidence. Other online resources, such as the National Heart, Lung, and Blood Institute, have outdated material emphasizing low-fat foods and indicating sweets are okay if they're "low-fat." We believe everything in moderation is key, and a healthy and balanced life is important. We believe sweets are okay in moderation, and it's unrealistic to give up forever something you love.

The newest research on DASH diet emphasizes cutting back on not only empty calories but empty carbs as well. Empty calories are calories derived from food that provide little or no nutritional benefit, such as candy and alcohol, and empty carbs are highly processed foods with a lot of added sugar and little to no nutritional value, such as starchy foods like breads and pastas. Also, the newest research on the DASH diet includes more protein and heart-healthy fats.

The reason why there is such success with the new DASH diet studies, such as improved blood pressure and sustainable, lasting weight loss, is because protein and fats allow you to feel full, whereas high carb intake leaves you feeling hungry in a shorter period of time. Fortunately for you, the newest research reveals that to maintain weight loss and have improved health, and more specifically, improved kidney outcomes, one must consume bulky, satisfying, satiating foods. This probably goes against what you've learned over the years when going on a diet.

---

4   National Heart, Lung, and Blood Institute, "DASH Eating Plan," US Department of Health and Human Services, Accessed January 12, 2018, https://www.nhlbi.nih.gov/health-topics/dash-eating-plan.

# What Is the DASH Diet?

Diets, for the past few decades, have been based on sugar-free (aka fake sugar), low-fat, frozen, microwavable meals, such as LeanCuisine or SmartOnes; meal replacements; and more glorified junk foods. The beauty of the DASH diet, and we will continue to emphasize this, is that it's not a diet—it's a lifestyle! A diet is short-term and usually results in gaining the weight back once you fall back into your old habits.

By embracing the DASH diet, we want you to learn behaviors that you can use for the rest of your life. We want you to learn that if you eat real, whole foods and consume reasonable portions, you'll never have to diet again. So many of our patients come in to the session admitting to having been chronic dieters their whole life. This includes yo-yo dieting, restricting, depriving, binging, and following every commercial diet in the book. After educating and counseling them on nutrition and encouraging them to eat a real, whole food, balanced diet, they see the results they always desired. The weight comes off slowly but sustainably, they feel good, they build confidence, and they make behavioral changes. All these results without a magic pill or feeling deprived. Changing your lifestyle takes time, and even if results don't come so quickly, they are lasting and maintainable. The DASH diet will put you on the road to your healthiest self yet.

Foods such as the following are emphasized in the newest DASH research:

- carbohydrates in the form of fruits and vegetables (high-fiber carbs)
- protein from either plants or animals
- heart-healthy fats such as avocadoes, nuts, and seeds

It's as simple as that: eat a balance of protein, fat, and carbs (nicknamed PFC). If you eat PFC at all of your meals, you'll be consuming a variety of nutrients and calories that will properly fuel you and satiate you, leading to reduced cravings and binge eating. Avoiding empty carb intake and fueling your body with necessary PFCs allows you to avoid the blood-sugar roller coaster that many Americans have been riding for far too long. Read about the blood-sugar roller coaster and the low-fat crisis beginning on page 42.

# What the Diet Requires of You

Not much is required of you besides small changes in your food choices, the desire for a healthier lifestyle and body, and some behavior modification (this is something ALL of us need!). Behavior modification is the action of taking small strides to replace negative eating behaviors with positive eating behaviors. An example of this is if you usually order an extra-large soda, replacing that behavior by ordering a medium soda. The next step would be to order a small soda and, ultimately, no soda. Or, rather than getting fries with a meal, replacing it with roasted veggies. There are many techniques to help you modify poor nutrition behaviors.

While this book will provide tips and tons of nutrition information, modifying your personal behaviors is ultimately in your hands. You have the power to get in touch with your mind and body, which will allow you to see what's causing you to make unhealthy choices. Once you can pinpoint the cause of unhealthy behaviors, you can work to change them.

## How to Modify Behaviors on the DASH Diet

First, try to understand what causes you to eat unhealthy. Do any of the following factors influence your eating patterns?
- Time of the day
- Emotions
- Certain activities, such as work parties
- Having company over or going out to dinner
- Habit
- Lack of nutrition knowledge
- Lack of a support system

Next, keep a food journal to better understand your eating habits and patterns. Write down what time of the day you are eating, how much you are eating, and how you feel. Then, write down behaviors you would like to change in one column. In the next column, write down a healthy behavior you can replace it with. See the chart below for some examples of poor nutrition behaviors you can replace with healthier ones. In the fourth example, try to come up with your own replacement behavior.

| Poor Nutrition Behaviors | Replace with Healthy Nutrition Behavior |
|---|---|
| I order an extra-large soda at restaurants. | I will order a medium soda. |
| I order fries as a side with my lunch daily. | I will order roasted potatoes with lunch. |
| I put six sugar packets in my coffee daily. | I will reduce the added sugar packets to four. |
| I eat three scoops of ice cream for dessert nightly. | You try to come up with a replacement behavior. |

For those who tend to overeat and have poor portion control:
- Designate one room for eating. Avoid eating in your bedroom, living room, and especially in front of the TV.
- Place just enough food on your plate for satisfaction (not to feel overwhelmingly full).
- Learn about proper portion sizes! Purchase a portion control plate and portion control lunch box (bento box) to help you in the beginning.
- Put leftovers away immediately.
- Portion out your meals in Tupperware.
- Ask others to support your efforts, especially when dining out.

If you have a good understanding of the importance of behavior modification, let's move on.

The DASH diet does not require:

- Special foods
- Purchase of prepackaged meals or meal-replacement shakes
- Hard-to-follow recipes
- Giving up your favorite foods
- Cutting out a macronutrient

The diet calls for, but does not require, the consumption of a certain number of daily servings from important food groups, depending on your recommended daily caloric needs. We understand that calorie counting and keeping track of food group intake may not be for everybody. And that's okay! Some people make the best food choices and healthy changes when they *aren't* counting calories and feeling overwhelmed with food tracking. Some people also feel discouraged when restricted to a certain number of calories per day. A lot of times, our patients tell us that if they're told to do something specific such as this, they'll do the exact opposite. That is why if counting calories is not something you're interested in or you know it won't aid in your success, you may skip over this part and head to Compare Your Current Eating Regimen to DASH on page 26. Calorie counting is not essential for your success on the DASH diet, as long as you're consuming proper portion sizes and healthful foods.

Your recommended daily calorie needs based on your activity level are shown in the chart on page 23. Activity levels are:

**Sedentary**—Light physical activity; day-to-day activities are your only physical activity (cleaning, food shopping, etc.).

**Moderately Active**—Walking about 1 to 3 miles per day, plus light weight-bearing activity.

**Active**—Walking more than 3 miles per day, plus weight-bearing activity multiple times per week for at least 15 minutes.

This is not set in stone, but rather a very general recommendation. If you are at a healthy weight, consume a specific number of calories per day, and your body responds well, by all means, continue with it.

## YOUR DAILY CALORIE NEEDS
### (CALORIES NEEDED FOR EACH ACTIVITY LEVEL)

|  | Age (years) | Female | Male |
|---|---|---|---|
| **Sedentary** Light physical activity; day-to-day activities are your only physical activity (cleaning, food shopping, etc.). | 19–30 | 2,000 | 2,400 |
| | 31–50 | 1,800 | 2,200 |
| | 51+ | 1,600 | 2,000 |
| **Moderately Active** Walking about 1 to 3 miles per day, plus light weight-bearing activity. | 19–30 | 2,000–2,200 | 2,600–2,800 |
| | 31–50 | 2,000 | 2,400–2,600 |
| | 51+ | 1,800 | 2,200–2,400 |
| **Active** Walking more than 3 miles per day, plus weight-bearing activity multiple times per week. | 19–30 | 2,400 | 3,000 |
| | 31–50 | 2,200 | 2,800–3,000 |
| | 51+ | 2,000–2,200 | 2,400–2,800 |

National Heart, Lung, and Blood Institute, "In Brief: Your Guide to Lowering Your Blood Pressure with DASH," Revised August, 2015, https://www.nhlbi.nih.gov/files/docs/public/heart/dash_brief.pdf.

# Serving Sizes and Calorie Counting

Your recommended calorie level depends on your age, gender, and activity level. These general guidelines allow you to put the amount of calories in different foods into perspective. For example, before paying attention to calories, you may have consumed a whole bag of chips (at a whopping 900 calories). After understanding your general daily calorie needs (for example, 1,800 daily calories), you may think twice next time about wasting half of your calories for the day on a bag of chips. Calories allow you to understand the importance of a serving size, portions, and how calorically dense a meal is.

Restaurants and food operations are now putting calories on their menus. If your dinner contains 1,800 calories, which is often the case with restaurant dinners, then you may feel more inclined to take half home or share it with a friend. There's no need to consume 1,800 calories in one sitting. So, even if you are uninterested in counting calories daily, understanding what your general intake should be will help you make wise food choices and be more mindful of portions.

The chart on page 25 demonstrates how many servings of each food group should be consumed per day based on your calorie needs. The different food groups covered are:

- **Vegetables**. These include such foods as arugula, broccoli, Brussels sprouts, carrots, cabbage, collard greens, green beans, green peas, kale, potatoes, radishes, spinach, sweet potatoes, and tomatoes.

- **Fruits**. These include apples, apricots, bananas, blueberries, cranberries, grapes, mangoes, oranges, pomegranate, peaches, strawberries, and watermelon.

- **Grains**. These include sprouted grain bread or sprouted grain tortillas, whole grain bread, brown rice pasta, whole wheat pasta, whole grain English muffins, muesli, oats, unsalted grain pretzels, and popcorn.

- **Milk/milk-alternative products**. These include cow's milk, rice milk, almond milk, coconut milk, hemp milk, half and half, yogurt, kefir, frozen yogurt, and cheese.

- **Meat, poultry, and fish,** which provide protein and magnesium. These include beef, pork, lamb, chicken, turkey, salmon, and swordfish. Note: Meat should be broiled, roasted, grilled, or poached; do not fry in oil.

- **Nuts and seeds**. These include almonds, chia seeds, black beans, flax seeds, hazelnuts, nut butter, mixed unsalted nuts, walnuts, sunflower seeds, kidney beans, lentils, and split peas.

- **Fats and oils**. These include butter, oils, mayonnaise, and salad dressing.

- **Sweets and added sugar**. These include sodas, candy, Jell-O, juices, cookies, and energy drinks.

# RECOMMENDED CALORIE LEVEL AND SERVINGS PER DAY

| Servings | Examples of Serving Sizes |
|---|---|
| **Vegetables**<br>nutrients provided: potassium, magnesium, fiber | |
| 4 or more (1,600 calories/day)<br>5 or more (2,000 calories/day)<br>6 or more (2,600 calories/day) | • 1 cup raw leafy green vegetables<br>• ½ cup raw or cooked vegetables |
| **Fruits**<br>nutrients provided: potassium, magnesium, fiber | |
| 3 (1,600 calories/day)<br>3–4 (2,000 calories/day)<br>4–5 (2,600 calories/day) | • 1 medium fruit (size of fist)<br>• ¼ cup dried fruit<br>• ½ cup fresh, frozen, or canned (drain and rinse well)<br>• ½ cup fruit juice (limit) |
| **Grains**<br>nutrients provided: fiber | |
| 4 (1,600 calories/day)<br>4–5 (2,000 calories/day)<br>5–6 (2,600 calories/day) | • 1 slice sprouted grain or whole grain bread<br>• 1 ounce dry cereal or muesli<br>• ½ cup hot cereal (oats)<br>• ½ cup cooked brown rice or pasta |
| **Milk/Milk-Alternative Products (this is not required)**<br>nutrients provided: calcium, protein | |
| 1–2 (1,000 calories/day)<br>2–3 (2,000 calories/day)<br>3–4 (2,600 calories/day) | • 1 cup (8 ounces) milk<br>• 1 cup yogurt<br>• 1.5 ounces cheese |
| **Meats, poultry, and fish**<br>nutrients provided: protein, magnesium | |
| 1–2 (1,000 calories/day)<br>2 (2,000 calories/day)<br>2–3 (2,600 calories/day) | • 3 ounce cooked meat, poultry, or fish<br>• 1 egg<br>• 2 egg whites |

| Servings | Examples of Serving Sizes |
|---|---|
| **Nuts, seeds, and legumes**<br>nutrients provided: magnesium, protein, fiber | |
| 1–2 *(1,600 calories/day)*<br>2–3 *(2,000 calories/day)*<br>3–4 *(2,600 calories/day)* | • ⅓ cup nuts<br>• 2 tablespoons nut butter<br>• 2 tablespoons seeds<br>• ½ cup cooked legumes (beans or peas) |
| **Fats and oils**<br>nutrients provided: omega-3 fatty acids | |
| 4 *(1,600 calories/day)*<br>5 *(2,000 calories/day)*<br>6 *(2,600 calories/day)* | • 1 teaspoon butter<br>• 1 teaspoon oil (olive, grapeseed, coconut)<br>• 1 tablespoon mayo (unrefined)<br>• 2 tablespoons salad dressing (minimal ingredients list) |
| **Sweets and added sugars (this is not required)** | |
| very limited *(1,600 calories/day)*<br>very limited *(2,000 calories/day)*<br>very limited *(2,600 calories/day)* | • 1 tablespoon sugar<br>• 1 tablespoon jelly or jam<br>• 1 cup (8 fluid ounces) sugar-sweetened beverage |

# Compare Your Current Eating Regimen to DASH

Fill out a daily food log to better understand what you're consuming throughout the day, how your recommended servings and portions compare to what you're eating, and how often you are exercising. This is a good way to track your progress and see how, over time, your eating habits and food choices are improving. I've included a blank food log on page 166 that you can copy and use multiple times. This should help you develop short-term and long-term goals for food choices and behaviors. On the next page is a filled-out breakfast entry:

| Date: 1/10/18 | | Number of Servings | | |
|---|---|---|---|---|
| Food (include serving size) | Sodium (mg) | Grains | Nuts, seeds, legumes | How do you feel? |
| Breakfast<br>1 piece Ezekiel Flaxseed bread | 200 | 1 | | I feel satisfied and energized. |
| 1 tablespoon almond butter | 150 | | 1 | |

The chart is helpful in pinpointing places you could improve. For example, you may realize you could be eating a healthier piece of bread or eating only half of the pasta you usually consume. Paying attention to serving size, or portion size, is essential to staying on track. And, of course, listening to your body and hunger cues. Asking, *"Am I actually hungry or am I just eating because I am bored?"* is a good step in being honest with yourself and recognizing hunger and fullness cues.

# DASH Diet in Sum

In sum, there are no gimmicks involved. You don't need to drink cabbage soup, eat only purple foods, or anything silly like that. It's not a diet that asks you to drastically alter your lifestyle, like a carb-limiting diet. Instead, we're going to introduce you to the healthy foundation that the DASH diet was based on—simple modifications that you can follow for the rest of your life. It's not a diet that you'll be talking about in five years saying, "Oh yeah, I followed that diet once. I lost weight but gained it all back." This is a diet that you will want to share with your friends and family. They will notice the change in your health and overall appearance, such as your skin, hair and nails, weight, and energy levels.

The DASH diet will help you rethink the way that you eat. And, before you know it, you won't have to focus so much on the small things, such as how much sodium is in this or how many bad ingredients are in that. You will learn over time and then just *know* what good foods fuel your body. You'll learn how to reduce the amount of sodium that you consume without losing the flavors you love, and you'll enjoy a variety of delicious foods that are rich in vitamins and nutrients that will help you get, and stay, healthy. With the DASH diet, there's no need to feel hungry or deprived: You'll enjoy lots of flavorful vegetables, fruits, whole grains, fish, poultry, and nuts.

The DASH diet was originally designed to lower blood pressure with diet and without the use of any medication. As nutritionists, we always say "use food as your first defense." It is common for doctors to prescribe you medication when you could cure yourself naturally with a healthy diet. For example, a patient that consumes a very-high-sugar diet is diagnosed with prediabetes, so immediately the doctor suggests going on Metformin. Why go on Metformin as your first line of defense when you can look at your diet, work with a dietitian, and make realistic lifestyle changes to lower your blood sugar and possibly prevent the need for medication the rest of your life?

Too many people are searching for quick fixes or taking whichever pill they've been told is necessary. Conditions such as prediabetes or prehypertension are warnings that should be taken seriously, and a plan of action must be developed. Getting diagnosed with one of these conditions doesn't mean you must run to get a prescription filled. This book will help you understand the direct connection nutrition has with your lab results, important organs, disease, and overall general health. (Please note, if you take medication to control high blood pressure, you should continue taking it. If you wish to stop taking it to lower your blood pressure naturally with a kidney-friendly diet, discuss this with your doctor.)

That being said, we admire the DASH diet simply because of the fact that it was originally designed to lower blood pressure with food and dietary changes. The first outcomes of research showed that the diet could lower blood pressure just as well as top-of-the-line blood pressure medications. Read that previous line again: It can lower blood pressure just as well as top-of-the-line medications.

Not to mention the added benefit that it's an effective solution to for sustainable weight loss, or losing weight and keeping it off. This is because when you're eating real, whole, nutritious foods, your body is happy, responds well, and can function properly without having to compensate for being fueled improperly. Think of your body like a car. Fuel it with what it needs (gas), and it'll run. Fuel it with what's not needed (water), and it simply will not run. Your body works the same way.

If you already have chronic kidney disease (CKD), you should speak with your doctor and dietitian before starting any new diets, as you may have certain dietary restrictions to consider. Consuming high potassium and phosphorous is not usually an issue in early stages of CKD, but lowering intake is usually recommended in stage 3 or stage 4.

The DASH diet should not be used by people on dialysis due to the high potassium and phosphorous content. Individuals on dialysis have special dietary needs that should be discussed with a registered dietitian. Nutrition for dialysis is discussed beginning on page 78.

*Chapter 3*

# DASH DIET AND YOUR KIDNEYS

The DASH in DASH diet stands for Dietary Approaches to Stop Hypertension. Hypertension is a word for high blood pressure, which makes the heart work extremely hard and increases the risk of cardiovascular disease, such as heart disease (the number one cause of death nationwide) and stroke (the third cause of death nationwide).

The DASH diet, recommended by the National Kidney Foundation and approved by the National Heart, Lung, and Blood Institute, the American Heart Association, and the Dietary Guidelines for Americans, resets your metabolism and improves your kidney's response to high blood pressure. The original DASH diet and variations of the DASH diet (such as this book) are proven to significantly reduce blood pressure in as quickly as two weeks.

The DASH diet is full of vitamins and nutrients, like potassium, magnesium, calcium, and tummy-happy fiber. Scientists believe the combination of these nutrients work together to lower blood pressure because they promote sodium and fluid release from the body, directly helping arteries dilate, relax, and become more flexible.

Managing your blood pressure through the DASH diet is the most important step you can take to protect your kidneys. High blood pressure is unhealthy even if it stays only slightly above the normal level of less than 120/80 millimeters of mercury (mm Hg). The more blood pressure rises above the normal level, the greater the health risk. High blood pressure, protein in the urine (proteinuria), and kidney stones are common kidney issues that damage the kidneys and speed kidney failure progression. DASH reduces blood pressure, reduces proteinuria, prevents kidney stones, and delays progression of kidney failure or damage.

Though it was originally designed to solely help prevent and treat high blood pressure, the DASH diet may help lower cholesterol, manage or lower your weight, prevent or manage type 2 diabetes, and also prevent osteoporosis, cancer, heart disease, and stroke.[5] More than just a diet, DASH is about learning to adopt healthy eating behaviors, choosing nutritious foods that will fuel your body, and replacing not-so-healthy staples with delicious but good-for-you options.

# Understanding Blood Pressure Numbers

Blood pressure is measured using two numbers. The upper number, systolic blood pressure, measures the pressure in your blood vessels and against your artery walls when your heart beats. The lower number, diastolic blood pressure, indicates how much pressure your blood is exerting against your artery walls while the heart is resting between beats. If the measurements are 120 systolic and 80 diastolic, the numbers would read "120/80 mm Hg."

They are both important numbers, but the top number (systolic) is often given more attention as a risk factor for cardiovascular disease for those over 50 years of age. Usually this number rises with age due to increasing hardness of arteries and the buildup of plaque from over the years. A proper diet can prevent both! The chart on the next page from the American Heart Association shows the systolic and diastolic blood pressure goals.

---

5    Mayo Clinic Staff, "DASH Diet: Healthy Eating to Lower Your Blood Pressure," Mayo Clinic, April 8, 2016, https://www.mayoclinic.org/healthy-lifestyle/nutrition-and-healthy-eating/in-depth/dash-diet/art-20048456.

| Blood Pressure Category | Systolic mm Hg (upper number) | | Diastolic mm HG (lower number) |
|---|---|---|---|
| Normal | less than 120 | and | less than 80 |
| Prehypertension | 120–139 | or | 80–89 |
| High Blood Pressure (hypertension) stage 1 | 140–159 | or | 90–99 |
| High Blood Pressure (hypertension) stage 2 | 160 or higher | or | 100 or higher |
| Hypertensive Crisis; emergency care needed | higher than 180 | or | higher than 110 |

Either elevated systolic or diastolic blood pressure may be used to make a diagnosis of high blood pressure. Also, the risk of death from ischemic heart disease and stroke doubles with every 20 mm Hg systolic or 10 mm Hg diastolic increase for people between the ages of 40 and 89.[6]

Ischemic heart disease is the term for heart issues caused by narrow arteries. When arteries narrow, less blood flow and oxygen reaches the heart muscle, which can lead to a heart attack. The symptoms usually include chest pain or discomfort. The synonyms for ischemic heart disease are coronary artery disease (CAD) and coronary heart disease.

A stroke is often referred to as a "brain attack." It occurs when blood flow to an area of the brain is cut off. Then, brain cells are deprived of oxygen and die off. When brain cells die during the stroke, memory and muscles controlled by those cells are lost.

As you can see, high blood pressure is dangerous. It makes your heart work too hard, hardens the walls of your arteries, can cause the brain to hemorrhage, and causes the kidneys to function poorly. Overall, high blood pressure can lead to heart and kidney disease as well as strokes. The good news is that blood pressure can be lowered simply by following the DASH diet. Maintaining a healthy weight, being physically active for *at least* 2

---

6 "Understanding Blood Pressure Readings," Heart.org, November 2017, http://www.heart.org/HEARTORG/Conditions/HighBloodPressure/KnowYourNumbers/ Understanding-Blood-Pressure-Readings_UCM_301764_Article.jsp#.WZMp-63Myt8.

hours and 30 minutes per week, and moderating alcohol consumption are important factors that also aid in lowering your blood pressure.

# First Rule of the DASH Diet: Ditch Table Salt

The first rule of the DASH diet is to ditch table salt. You can avoid table salt simply by eating unrefined, whole foods, such as fruit, vegetables, eggs, beans, legumes, meat, poultry, and fish, which are the basic foods in the DASH diet. Removing processed foods from your diet, such as foods found in cans, boxes, and in the middle aisles of the grocery store, is one of the easiest ways to decrease table salt intake.

This doesn't mean ditch all salt for the rest of your life. That is unrealistic, and your body *needs* salt. Be mindful that when you increase your water intake, you lose salt, an essential nutrient. A good rule of thumb is for every 10 glasses of water you consume, ingest half a teaspoon of good-quality, mineral-containing salt, such as pink Himalayan or Celtic sea salt. Table salt differs from naturally occurring salt, a precious element that used to be a highly valued form of currency. Unless you're on a fluid restriction, these varieties are not the enemy, even though we have been taught that.

While it's true that salt binds to water in the bloodstream and raises blood pressure, it should not be demonized completely, as not all salts are created equally. Inferior to the quality, unrefined, untouched salts, table salt is chemically processed, bleached, and may contain added chemicals such as ammonia or aluminum. Aluminum consumption is highly toxic to the body. Prevalent in the food supply, it has been linked to neurodegenerative disorders, such as Alzheimer's and dementia.

If you eat whole, unprocessed foods most of the time and add reasonable amounts of quality salt to your food, it will not harshly impact your health as table salt does. Rather, natural salt provides your body with at least 60 minerals vital to organ function, including calcium, iodine, potassium, magnesium, and iron. Moreover, it contains triple the amount of potassium per serving than normal salt! Remember that potassium is one of the minerals that works to lower blood pressure in the body.

The issue with table salt is that all of its minerals, except for sodium and chloride, are stripped during the refining process. (Refining is never good. The more you eat foods in their natural form, the better.) Table salt is more damaging than the two salts mentioned above because it interferes with your body's natural sodium and potassium balance. Understand that sodium and potassium work together to affect blood pressure and heart disease risk. In a study involving 3,000 participants who were 30 to 54 years old and had prehypertension, researchers collected urine intermittently during 24-hour periods. One trial was a period of 18 months and the other 36 months. The urinary levels of sodium and potassium were compared with subsequent cardiovascular diseases in the 10- to 15-year follow-ups. The results showed a significant increase in the risk of cardiovascular disease with higher ratios of sodium to potassium. These results support the fact that lowering dietary sodium while increasing potassium intake can reduce the incidence of cardiovascular disease. Overall, the higher sodium-to-potassium ratio was a stronger indicator of increased risk among participants in the study than levels of sodium or potassium alone. This means getting your intake of potassium up is just as important as lowering your sodium intake!

Table salt only contains sodium (Na) and chloride (Cl). According to the *American Journal of Clinical Nutrition*, a diet high in sodium chloride (NaCl) can raise blood pressure as the kidneys retain NaCl together with high intake. Also, a high-potassium diet reduces the rise of blood pressure caused by a high NaCl diet, whereas low or normal potassium intake is related to increased blood pressure.

## Our Ancestors and Sodium Intake

Prehistorically, humans and mammals evolved in a low-NaCl environment, so the harmful effects of a high-NaCl diet are not really unexpected. Thousands of years ago when our ancestors gathered and hunted food, potassium was abundant and sodium was scarce. This is known as the Paleolithic Era, which is the basis of the modern and popular Paleo diet.

In this time, fruits, vegetables, leaves, and other plants were widely abundant and provided a wealth of potassium in the diet.

Ever wonder why people hold onto sodium, or retain water, in their body? Or why consuming a lot of sodium causes your body to gain temporary fluid weight? Well, the scarcity of sodium in these times is reflected in this mechanism. In some people, especially those with kidney dysfunction, hypertension, and heart disease, the kidneys hold onto sodium and further complicate diseases. When you consume sodium, your body is trying to maintain the proper sodium and water concentration. Sodium today is cheap, prevalent in the food supply, hidden in processed foods, inexpensive, and widely abundant in the SAD, so high blood pressure and high sodium intake is not unexpected either.

Our modern diet goes against the evolutionary forces that allowed mammals to adapt well to a low-sodium diet. Evidence suggests that a high-NaCl diet can cause an increase in mortality, which can be defined as the relative incidence of death within a particular group categorized according to age or some other factor.

## Salt and Potassium in the Standard American Diet

Without question, the SAD is high in processed table salt found in many packaged foods, such as cookies, chips, and breads. On average, Americans consume about 3,300 milligrams of sodium per day, which is almost 1.5 teaspoons of salt. This amount is way beyond the recommended amount of 2,300 milligrams per day for healthy people and 1,500 milligrams per day for middle-aged and older individuals, African Americans, and those with high blood pressure. Approximately 2,600 milligrams of potassium are consumed per day compared to the recommended 4,700 milligrams or more. (Here we are stressing the importance of potassium, again.)

According to nationwide food consumption surveys, potassium is a nutrient Americans don't get enough of, along with vitamin D. Deficiencies in these nutrients are associated with an increased risk of chronic diseases. Potassium is an underconsumed nutrient in the SAD to the extent that in 2016, the FDA required food manufacturers to not only include potassium on the Nutrition Facts label, but the actual amounts in addition to the % daily value (%DV). Manufacturers must comply with the changes to the Nutrition Facts label by July 26, 2018. Manufacturers with less than $10 million in annual food sales will have an additional year to make the changes. Some food companies, such as KIND, have already made the final changes to their label. See Get to Know Your Nutrition Facts Label on page 98 for information on how to read the Nutrition Facts label.

# Restoring the Balance with DASH

Blood pressure experts previously believed that simply reducing sodium was the key to restoring blood pressure. We now know that in order to restore blood pressure, you must restore the healthy balance between sodium and potassium intake. Ideally, potassium-to-sodium intake should be 2:1. This means consuming twice as much potassium than sodium is ideal, and, as you know, this isn't what most people consuming the SAD follow.

The kidneys respond to excess sodium by excreting it in urine. However, this also removes potassium. Think of sodium and potassium as a dynamic duo. These two elements go hand in hand—an imbalance wreaks havoc in the body. When potassium levels are low, which is very common in Americans, the body tries to hold onto it because it's unsure when it'll get more of the necessary nutrient. This is similar to the concept of people consuming very-low-calorie diets and wondering why they can't lose weight. Your body is deprived of the proper nutrition and calories and is unsure when it'll get refueled, so it holds onto what it has and is put into starvation mode. This idea is related to the car example. If there is no gas in your tank, your car won't run. If your body is not fueled with enough food, your metabolism is slowed down in an attempt to conserve energy. Your body has mechanisms to stay alive, and this is one of them. With low potassium intake, your body also holds onto the sodium. Your body can get rid of sodium by increasing potassium intake.

A report from the Trials of Hypertension Prevention (sponsored by the National Heart, Lung, and Blood Institute) stresses the importance of balancing these two minerals. Nancy Cook, a biostatistician at Harvard-affiliated Brigham and Women's Hospital states, "Our study suggests that just lowering sodium, or just raising potassium, won't be nearly as effective for fighting hypertension or heart disease as doing both together."

## Bringing Sodium Up Again

The DASH diet makes it easier to eat less sodium because the foods emphasized the most—fruits and vegetables—are naturally lower in sodium than many other foods. Your sodium limit is either 2,300 milligrams or 1,500 milligrams if you are following a lower-sodium DASH diet. Typical table salt consists of sodium chloride, which is 40% sodium.

Below shows the measurements of sodium in typical white table salt:

¼ teaspoon = 575 mg sodium

½ teaspoon = 1,150 mg sodium

¾ teaspoon = 1,725 mg sodium

1 teaspoon = 2,300 mg sodium

One teaspoon of sodium will put you at your sodium restriction for the day. It may sound like 1 teaspoon of sodium is easy to use, but don't worry, sodium is not used as freely as sugar. It's very, very unlikely you're adding 1 teaspoon of sodium to your meals. A general guideline is to select foods with 140 milligrams of sodium or less per serving. When a food label reads "low-sodium," it will contain less than 140 milligrams per serving, and "very low-sodium" will contain less than 35 milligrams of sodium per serving. Foods with more than 300 milligrams of sodium per serving are not ideal. Remember, if you eat two servings rather than one, you are getting double the amount of sodium. Also, "unsalted" or "no added salt" foods can still have naturally occurring sodium, so always read the Nutrition Facts label to confirm, regardless of the claims on the front of the package.

# Salty Six

The American Heart Association warns of surprisingly (or not so!) high sodium levels in six common foods. While potato chips and the salt shaker take most of the blame for hypertension, there are plenty of other foods contributing to excess sodium consumption. What's more, what is *already* in the food products is also to blame for excess sodium intake, not only what we are *adding* to food.

**1. Breads and rolls.** These are eaten several times a day, but little thought is given to their sodium content. One piece of bread can have as much as 230 milligrams of sodium. While this doesn't sound like much, if you're eating toast at breakfast and a sandwich for dinner, that's already 690 milligrams of sodium. That is almost half of the recommended sodium intake for most adults.

*What can you do?* Purchase low-sodium breads. For example, Ezekiel 4:9 contains 0 milligrams of sodium in one slice of bread. Yes, absolutely no sodium. The Ezekiel 4:9 English muffins contain 150 milligrams in one muffin (which could be used as a burger bun), whereas a typical hamburger bun has 250 milligrams of sodium. Typically, you should aim to choose a bread that is less than 80 milligrams per slice. You can also make super-nutritious homemade breads with or without reduced-sodium baking soda.

**2. Cold cuts and cured meats.** These include, but are not limited to, bacon, ham, sausages, and pepperoni. A 2-ounce serving of deli meat can contain up to 800 milligrams of sodium.

*What can you do?* Look for low-sodium varieties of deli meat, fresh meats, fish, and turkey bacon. Always compare food labels of different products to choose the one with the lowest amount of sodium. Choose foods not packaged in a sodium solution.

**3. Sandwiches or burgers.** It's never a good idea to order a sandwich or burger from a restaurant for the sole fact that it will inevitably be high in sodium due to the bread, sauces, cheese, and meat. For example, the spicy Italian sandwich from Subway contains 1,550 milligrams of sodium.

*What can you do?* Opt for more veggie-based sandwiches. For example, the Veggie Delite at Subway contains only 280 milligrams of sodium! You could also order half a sandwich with a side salad.

**4. Pizza.** One slice of pizza with toppings, especially meat toppings, can contain more than half of your daily recommended dietary sodium.

*What can you do?* Add veggie toppings to your pizza or try making a homemade pizza so you know exactly how much sodium is going into it.

**5. Chicken.** While chicken is a healthy meat option, be mindful of the sodium content. The sodium amounts will vary based on preparation methods. For example, a 4-ounce serving of rotisserie chicken can contain up to 600 milligrams of sodium.

*What can you do?* Try to always purchase fresh chicken breast, leg, thigh, or any cut you prefer. It's always best to season meat yourself. The healthiest ways to cook chicken are the following: baking, grilling, steaming, or stir-frying.

**6. Canned soup.** While soup can be a delicious way to get in a large amount of nutrients and veggies, a serving from canned soup can get you close to your daily sodium limit. For example, Campbell's Homestyle Chicken Noodle Soup contains 940 milligrams of sodium per cup.

*What can you do?* Compare labels to find lower-sodium varieties and always look for "low-sodium" on the front label. Making your own soup in a pot, slow cooker, or pressure cooker is the best option. You can make a large batch of soup and have it ready for the week or freeze it in Tupperware for later use.

# Tips to Reduce Sodium Intake

Salt restriction is sometimes referred to as No-Added-Salt, or NAS. As you've learned, sodium isn't only found in the salt shaker. Rather, it's hidden everywhere, especially in processed, shelf-stable foods. Sodium can almost always be found in processed foods from cans and boxes. Sodium is added to preserve the food, which allows it to sit on shelves for years (this isn't good; your food shouldn't outlive your goldfish). Unfortunately, it's also in fresh foods, because it's part of their composition, such as pickles, olives, garlic, onions, and milk. Sodium can also be found in canned vegetables because they're packaged in a salt solution.

Some chemical ingredients also contain sodium, such as the following: monosodium glutamate or MSG, sodium saccharin, sodium phosphates, sodium citrate, sodium caseinate, sodium benzoate, and sodium nitrite. Again, consuming real, fresh whole foods completely eliminates the issue of worrying about additives and preservatives.

From the grocery aisles to your dinner table, sodium has plenty of opportunities to make its way into your body. It is up to you to make choices that'll reduce your sodium intake. It may take time for your taste buds to adjust to a lower-sodium diet, but they will. This concept is similar to people focusing on reducing sugar intake. One cannot go from adding 8 teaspoons of sugar into their coffee to 1 teaspoon the next day. It takes time, patience, and gradual steps to reach such goals. Once the adjustment is made, you'll feel great and do your body a huge favor. Once people reach their goal, often they will report how they don't know how they previously added "so much salt" or "so much sugar," and how they will never go back to it. Here are some tips to decrease sodium intake:

- Be mindful of salt substitutes. Many salt substitutes contain large amounts of potassium, which may need to be avoided. A safe salt-free substitute is Mrs. Dash seasonings, which offers a variety of herb blends to heighten the flavor of your foods.

- Use herbs, spices, and aromatic vegetables. Herbs and spices provide savory additions to enhance natural flavors without the salt. Aromatic vegetables, such as onions, peppers, and garlic, also impart wonderful flavor without the salt.

- Flavor food with fruit. Fruit, especially citrus, such as lemon or lime juice, bring freshness to any dish.

- Read food labels. Be sure to check the labels before purchasing anything, and take special note sodium content—even if foods don't taste salty, they certainly can be.

- Limit processed foods as much as possible. These include frozen dinners, frozen pizzas, canned soups, and other items that come in cans or boxes in the middle aisles of the supermarket. Choose and purchase soups, beans, and other canned goods that read "low-sodium." Prepare your own food and freeze for later use.

- Frozen packaged foods, especially in sauces, tend to contain high amounts of sodium. Try buying plain frozen foods, such as fruits and vegetables.

- If you are eating an item that is processed with high sodium, eat half. Bulk up the rest of the meal with microwavable frozen veggies. This is a quick and easy way to reduce sodium intake and get those veggies in.

- Use cut-up fruits and veggies as snacks. Pair them with a healthy fat or protein source, such as almond butter, hummus, or guacamole.

- Choose unsalted nuts and seeds. Flavor them by adding spices (such as curry) and roasting them in the oven or on a pan with coconut oil.

- Skip supermarket herbs and start an herb garden on your kitchen counter. You will be surprised at how much flavor and aroma they have compared to dried supermarket versions.

- Remove the salt shaker from your table.

- Aim for foods that contain 5% or less of the daily value of sodium. Foods with 20% or more daily value of sodium are considered high, such as baked goods, certain cereals, soups, and soy sauces.

- When dining out, ask how the food is prepared. These dishes or ingredients normally indicate high-sodium content: cured meats, soy sauce, broth, and sauce-based dishes. Ask that the meal be prepared without added salt, monosodium glutamate (MSG), or other salt-containing ingredients. Also request condiments and dressings on the side and use as little as possible, such as ketchup and spicy mayo. You can always bring your own, too! Move the salt shaker out of your reach and possibly bring your own Mrs. Dash seasoning or other salt-free seasonings.

# The Blood Sugar Roller Coaster

During nutrition counseling sessions, we make a point to discuss the blood sugar roller coaster with every single patient. We think it's crucial for you to understand this, too. Blood sugar control is not just essential for those with diabetes, but for anybody who wants to fight sugar cravings, keep off extra weight, and keep up energy levels. When you eat a carbohydrate, regardless of the source (bread, pasta, rice, candy, cookies, muffins, soda, and even fruits or vegetables), it turns into sugar in your bloodstream. Fruits and vegetables, of course, have necessary vitamins, minerals, and fiber, so they're excellent carb choices. Regardless, after consuming a carb, your blood sugar levels spike, and insulin, a fat-storing hormone, is released. Insulin allows sugar to get into your cells and out of the bloodstream, reducing your blood sugar levels. As you know, in almost all circumstances, what goes up must come down. Thus, when you have a diet high in carbs, there is a cycle of spikes and drops in blood sugar levels *all day long*.

By including healthy fats and protein in your diet, you slow down the absorption of carbohydrates and, ultimately, keep blood sugar levels stable. Blood sugar stability is not only beneficial for your waistline, but also to reduce or reverse type 2 diabetes, reduce triglycerides, improve HDL cholesterol, lower LDL cholesterol, reduce cravings, stabilize moods, and much more.

If you have already consumed enough of the carbs your body needs, which is often the case in the high-carb SAD, then the sugar is stored as fat since it cannot be used for energy. See, carbs became the focus of meals once people began low-fat diets. And what happened? The extra carbs are stored as fat, contributing to weight gain and other chronic diseases.

With kidney disease, it's especially important to control your blood sugar, especially if CKD resulted from diabetes. Good blood sugar control can help slow down the progression of kidney disease in people with diabetes. Your kidneys are forced to work overtime to filter and absorb the excess sugar. Thus, poor blood glucose can damage your kidneys and other parts of your body, such as your eyes and feet. High levels of blood glucose may also increase your thirst, making it difficult to limit fluid intake. Excessive thirst is called polydipsia. It occurs when excess sugar builds up in the blood and the kidneys can't keep up. When the kidneys can't filter all the sugar, it is excreted in urine, taking along fluids from tissues.

One way to keep blood sugars under control is to plan meals and snacks at similar times each day. Also, stick to eating approximately the same amount of servings, or grams, of carbs for each meal. The same goes for snacks—if you're eating a piece of fruit and handful of nuts, try to have the same carb content at the next snack. This will keep your blood sugars nice and stable. Snacks are important to help manage your blood glucose levels.

# Anemia and CKD

As discussed in Chapter 1, the kidneys have many important roles in the body, from maintaining homeostasis to filtering the blood and flushing waste products in urine. Another is to produce a hormone called erythropoietin. Erythropoietin prompts the bone marrow to make red blood cells. Red blood cells then carry oxygen throughout the body to maintain healthy oxygen levels in the body's tissues and organs.

You may know that iron-deficiency anemia is a condition in which the body has fewer red blood cells than normal. The lack of oxygenated red blood cells causes the following signs and symptoms:

- Weakness
- Fatigue
- Headaches
- Problems concentrating
- Paleness
- Dizziness
- Difficulty breathing or shortness of breath
- Chest pain

Anemia commonly occurs in people with CKD and tends to worsen as CKD progresses. This is simply because when kidney dysfunction is present, they are unable to make enough erythropoietin. Thus, the bone marrow makes fewer red blood cells, depriving the body of the oxygen it needs. Complications of anemia in those with CKD include heart issues, commonly irregular heartbeat or fast heartbeat, enlargement of muscles in the heart, and heart failure.

Anemia could begin to develop in the early stages of CKD, which is when someone has approximately 20% to 50% of normal kidney function.[7] (See the stages of chronic kidney disease on page 11.) In stage 5 of CKD, which is renal failure, the prevalence of anemia is 53.4%.[8] One has renal failure when they need a kidney transplant or dialysis in order to live.

If you are on dialysis, such as hemodialysis, you could be anemic due to blood loss. Consuming inadequate amounts of certain nutrients, such as iron, vitamin B12, and folic acid can also cause anemia. These nutrients are necessary for red blood cells to make hemoglobin, a protein in the red blood cells that is responsible for carrying oxygen.

If blood tests indicate that kidney disease is likely the cause of anemia, injections of genetically engineered erythropoietin can be used as treatment. Often, iron supplements will be used to raise red blood cell count to prevent the need for red blood cell transfusions. B12 and folic acid may also be recommended supplements. Your doctor or dietitian will discuss your individual supplement recommendations with you. Never take advice from the internet or a book because supplementation should be individualized to your needs.

## Anemia Nutrition Therapy

It's important to include iron, vitamin B12, or folic acid in the diet if anemia is caused by inadequate intake of any of these nutrients. However, some of these foods are high in sodium or phosphorous (nutrients those with CKD may be limiting). Be sure to read food labels or find out the amount of these nutrients in specific foods.

Iron from meat, fish, and poultry is best absorbed by the body, compared to iron from plant sources. Also, consuming foods high in vitamin

---

7  "Anemia in Chronic Kidney Disease," National Institute of Diabetes and Digestive and Kidney Diseases, July 1, 2014, https://www.niddk.nih.gov/health-information/kidney-disease/chronic-kidney-disease-ckd/anemia.

8  Melissa E. Stauffer and Tao Fan, "Prevalence of Anemia in Chronic Kidney Disease in the United States," PloS One, January 2, 2014, doi:https://doi.org/10.1371/journal.pone.0084943.

C, such as citrus juice and fruits, melons, dark green leafy vegetables, and potatoes, along with iron-rich foods, helps your body better absorb the iron. Limit coffee and tea when eating iron-rich foods because they can decrease the absorption of iron. Most importantly, limit milk intake or do not have milk when eating iron-rich foods, as the casein in milk makes it harder for the body to absorb iron.

The table below shows some foods that provide at least 1 to 2 milligrams of iron per serving. The recommended quantities of iron are the following:

- 11 milligrams for males 14 to 18 years old
- 15 milligrams for females 14 to 18 years old
- 8 milligrams for males 19 to 51+ years old
- 18 milligrams for females 19 to 50 years old
- 8 milligrams for females 51+ years old
- Pregnant females between the ages of 14 and 50 should have 27 milligrams, and lactating women should have 9 to 10 milligrams.

## IRON LEVELS OF SELECTED FOODS

| Food | Serving Size | Iron |
|------|-------------|------|
| Breakfast cereals fortified with 100% Daily Value of iron | 1 serving according to Nutrition Facts label | 18mg |
| Oysters | 3 ounces | 8mg |
| Spirulina | 1 ounce | 8mg |
| White beans | 1 cup | 8mg |
| Liver | 3 ounces | 4mg |
| Lentils | ½ cup | 3mg |
| Spinach, cooked | ½ cup | 3mg |
| Tofu | ½ cup | 3mg |
| Dark chocolate | 1 ounce | 3mg |
| Black beans | ½ cup | 2mg |

## IRON LEVELS OF SELECTED FOODS

| Food | Serving Size | Iron |
|------|-------------|------|
| Cashews | 1 ounce (18 nuts) | 2mg |
| Sardines | 3 ounces | 2mg |
| Chickpeas | ½ cup | 2mg |

Source: National Institutes of Health, Office of Dietary Supplements. https://ods.od.nih.gov/factsheets/Iron-HealthProfessional

# Vitamin D and Kidney Function

Vitamin D is crucial for several functions in the body. Be sure to consume enough food sources of vitamin D, as it's one of the most common deficiencies in America. Excellent vitamin-rich food sources include sardines, salmon, mackerel, tuna, eggs, and mushrooms. The best non-food source of vitamin D is sunlight!

Vitamin D is activated and modified by the kidney. Once activated, it stimulates the uptake of calcium from food. It is also important for the maintenance of healthy bones and helps regulate the response of the immune system to infection.

Healthy kidneys play a role in converting inactive vitamin D into the active form. When kidneys begin to fail, they can no longer activate vitamin D. Active vitamin D helps balance the amount of calcium and phosphorous in the body. It controls the absorption of them from food and regulates the parathyroid hormone (PTH). PTH is secreted by the parathyroid glands, located near the thyroid glands in the neck. With kidney failure, the parathyroid gland mistakenly senses a loss of calcium in the blood and produces excess PTH. This tells the body to take calcium out of the bones and put it in the bloodstream.

Excess calcium in the bloodstream causes a myriad of health issues. Calcium can deposit in soft tissues, and these calcifications are irreversible. If the heart becomes calcified, there can be a reduction in blood flow, causing a heart attack. Also, lung calcification can cause difficulty breathing. Lastly, joint calcification can be extremely painful. Excess PTH may cause secondary hyperparathyroidism, resulting in bone pain, weak bones, and easy fractures. Unfortunately, those with kidney failure are largely at risk for this.

# DASH Diet and Kidney Stones

Kidney stones are linked to a diet high in processed fructose, which is the sugar from fruit or honey, as well as other sugars. This is because sugar disrupts mineral relationships. For example, it interferes with calcium and magnesium absorption. If you're a soda drinker, be aware that the phosphoric acid in soda acidifies your urine and promotes stone formation. The dietary guidelines for kidney stones include eating fewer high-oxalate foods, increasing the amount of dietary calcium, limiting vitamin C consumption, drinking the right amount of fluids daily, not consuming excess protein, and limiting sodium. High-oxalate foods include spinach, bran flakes, rhubarb, beets, potato chips, French fries, nuts, and nut butters. Most plant foods have some oxalate, so it is not necessary to cut out foods that have some oxalates.

Diets that are high in fruits and vegetables increase urinary citrate. Citrate is an inhibitor of calcium stone formation. Calcium stones are the most common type of kidney stones. This means that high vegetable and fruit intake will decrease your risk for kidney stones!

Consumption of a DASH-style diet was independently associated with a decreased risk of kidney stone formation in three large cohort studies performed by the *Journal of the American Society of Nephrology*, the leading kidney journal in the world. Although diets high in oxalates and vitamin C, such as the DASH diet, usually contribute to kidney stone formation, the study showed that people who consume higher amounts of calcium, potassium, and magnesium and less sodium, in addition to the oxalates and vitamin C, had a lower risk of kidney stone development. This means despite the high intake of oxalates and vitamin C in the DASH diet, the risk of kidney stone development is reduced. Also, a study in the *New England Journal of Medicine* found that diets with moderate to high calcium content and low animal protein and sodium intake can decrease the risk of calcium stone recurrence by 51%. Overall, this shows that a DASH diet rich in vegetables, fruits, and whole grains not only lowers blood pressure, but can reduce the risk of kidney stones. These are two important factors to prevent or delay kidney disease risk.

# How Low-Fat Made Us Fat

Fat is essential to your health. It gives you energy, helps you store energy in case you get sick and need "back up," and helps make more nutrients in your food available for your body to use. But some fats are good, and some are bad. Keep in mind, processed foods are usually created with damaging fats, such as trans fats. Man-made foods, foods not made by nature, are usually to blame for health issues, and are inflammatory.

The original DASH diet recommended low fat intake. However, the low-fat ideology never really had any scientific evidence supporting why it was necessary. More and more people today are realizing how low-fat ("lite," "skinny," "fat-free" products and foods) never really worked or were beneficial to our health. In fact, as this diet approach became popular, heart disease and other nutrition-related diseases skyrocketed. This is mainly due to the fact that when people consume low-fat foods, they increase their consumption of processed carbs and added sugar. Also, food companies need their products to taste good despite the loss of fat, so they almost always replace that removed fat with sugar.

Researchers at the University of California, San Francisco Benioff's Children's Hospital Oakland Research Institute (CHORI) conducted a randomized controlled trial to test how substituting a full-fat DASH diet versus the original low-fat DASH diet would affect blood pressure and important lab values such as LDL and HDL cholesterol levels. Keep in mind, the high-fat DASH diet includes an increase in fats and a reduction in carbohydrate, or sugar, intake. Published in the *American Journal of Clinical Nutrition*, the results were astonishing. The researchers found that the higher fat DASH diet not only lowered blood pressure to the same extent as the original DASH diet, but also reduced triglycerides and didn't significantly raise LDL cholesterol, the "bad cholesterol."

Just like cholesterol, fat is essential for every cell in our body, as it coats all cell membranes. Fat also has many other roles, such as being a key player in our nervous system, brain function, skin integrity, vitamin and mineral absorption, metabolism and brain function support, and healthy hormone production. It even has healing and immune-boosting properties. In other words, good fats can help rev up your metabolism, help you focus, balance hormones, and make skin glow!

Fats allow us to feel satiated (or full) and they decrease craving—unlike sugar and high-carb foods. Fat has unnecessarily been deemed a "bad" food. But how many people do you know who went on a low-fat diet and succeeded? It's not realistic, because fat is a macronutrient. The other two macronutrients are carbs and protein. We must include all three macronutrients in our diets to support a healthy, complete, and balanced diet. Hint: Carbohydrates in the form of fruits and veggies are the most beneficial because they are full of fiber, vitamins, and minerals. The DASH diet really emphasizes fruit and veggie consumption.

As with all other foods, there are healthy fats and not-so-healthy fats that are harmful to your body, as not all fats are created equally.

## The Truth About Cholesterol

Most of us have been led to believe that cholesterol, along with fat, is the culprit behind heart disease. Most of our life, that's what we've been taught, right? Unfortunately, this claim never had evidence to back it up, and we were listening to the wrong advice for *years*. Also, a lot of this advice was fueled by research studies sponsored by companies who wanted the outcome to be swayed to their benefit. In fact, cholesterol protects us from heart disease, atherosclerosis, and stroke.

First, you must understand what cholesterol is and what it does for the body. Cholesterol is a fat-like substance produced by the liver and most of our cells. You need cholesterol to survive. It doesn't dissolve in water, so it waterproofs our cells and holds them together, meaning cholesterol is vital to cell function. It provides the structure, stiffness, and stability cells need. Cholesterol is mostly prevalent in the brain and nervous system. That is why a mother's breast milk is 60% cholesterol; it is necessary for development of an infant's brain and nervous system. Cholesterol works to create neurotransmitters such as serotonin and dopamine, and it helps them reach their receptors. Also, hormones in the body, such as testosterone and estrogen, are made from cholesterol. Likewise, corticosteroids, the hormones that protect the body from stress and protect immune system function, are made from cholesterol.

Another function of cholesterol is to produce vitamin D. Vitamin D is a *very* common deficiency in the SAD—so much so that approximately 80% of the patients we've seen have been deficient in their yearly bloodwork. Cholesterol also creates bile salts, which break down carbs, fat, and protein. What's more, it helps maintain the intestinal wall, protecting the body from inflammation.

Overall, cholesterol is very protective of your immune system and works to heal the damage caused by inflammation. When inflammation occurs, cholesterol rushes over to repair and protect cells and membranes from damage. Cholesterol levels may increase when your body is fighting inflammation that stems from the overconsumption of sugar and processed carbohydrates. This inflammation is caused by overconsumption of sugar and processed carbohydrates. So, we've been blaming cholesterol for causing heart disease but it's actually been coming to the rescue to heal us! What's more, only a very small amount of the cholesterol you eat is found in your blood. This means dietary cholesterol does not equal high blood cholesterol.

Lowering high cholesterol with medicine, such as statins, will not heal the underlying problem. This is why it's always important to understand the root cause of any issue you may have.

## LDL Cholesterol's Bad Rap

As you may have learned from getting bloodwork done, there are two types of cholesterol: HDL and LDL cholesterol. LDL has a bad reputation, just as fats do, but it's all changing! During dietetic school, LDL cholesterol being the "bad" cholesterol was on many of the exams. Yes, dietetic school textbooks are outdated. The truth is, we as health professionals, and you as consumers, have been given an oversimplified view of LDL cholesterol.

To increase your nutritional knowledge, it's important to know that there are two types of LDL cholesterol, made up of two different particle sizes, and it shouldn't automatically be deemed the "bad cholesterol."

Type A can be remembered as big and puffy (these are healthy and healing). Type B is made up of small, dense particles (these are harmful and cause inflammation). Type B can readily enter compromised arterial walls, squeeze through the lining of your arteries, and fuel the inflammatory process if they oxidize, whereas the large puffy ones don't do this. So, when your doctor tells you that you have high LDL cholesterol, do not be alarmed. You have to know the whole makeup and find out the LDL particle size. If your doctor refuses to do this, you can get a Nuclear Magnetic Resonance (NMR) Lipoprofile test. (Visit walkinlab.com to learn more.)

So, what does this mean for you? The DASH diet? Your kidneys? It means we're not going to tell you to consume low-fat milk, low-fat cheese, or *anything* low-fat. Full-fat foods (olive oil, nuts, seeds, avocados) are a key component of a healthy and balanced diet. This is why, and you may find it hard to believe, we're not another book demanding you to consume low-fat foods. Fats have seriously made a comeback from their horrible reputation in the '90s—and for good reason.

*Chapter 4*

# DASH DIET GUIDELINES FOR KIDNEY HEALTH

Your kidneys are responsible for filtering body fluids, excreting waste, and much more. When your kidneys aren't functioning properly, waste and fluid from food and liquids you consume can build up in your body. This is why certain nutrients must be limited—to reduce the amount of waste in your blood.

In simpler terms, processing certain nutrients can become too difficult for your body, which can be lead to toxicity if you don't follow your prescribed diet properly. It can be intimidating when your doctor or dietitian tells you to reduce your intake of certain nutrients, such as sodium, phosphorous, potassium, and sometimes fluids or protein. However, it is crucial to follow your individual dietary advice because waste and fluid built up in your body can cause other health problems, especially with your heart and bones.

In this chapter, we're going to list what foods contain these nutrients so you have easy, go-to lists of foods to reduce or avoid. This will come in handy, especially when grocery shopping or choosing what to eat at a restaurant. It can be discouraging when you're told to limit your intake of certain foods, but we'll review how to easily cut back on these foods and offer safe substitutes so that you can enjoy eating without feeling restricted or deprived.

Your prescribed renal diet will help sustain kidney function and delay total kidney failure, so it's important to follow it to the best of your ability. The strictness of your meal plan depends on the specific renal diet plan your doctor or registered dietitian has prescribed you. The *amount* of food you consume is just as important as the type of food you consume, so try your hardest to stick with the portion sizes recommended by your doctor or dietitian. Eating more than the serving size for a moderate or low-nutrient food will make it a high-nutrient food. We cannot suggest what specific portion sizes to consume because that is an individualized recommendation based on your specific health goals and needs, but we will discuss general portion sizes. Limiting certain foods, as recommended, can truly reduce kidney disease progression.

Remember that if your diet is limited in certain foods, it's important to consume adequate calories. Consuming enough calories throughout the day is necessary to prevent muscle breakdown and weight loss.

# Nutrients and Kidney Health

As we've discussed, you'll need to be mindful of your intake of foods that contain salt, unhealthy fats, protein, and certain minerals, some of which are the building blocks of your body and essential for functioning. But, as they say, you can have too much of a good thing, especially when these things hurt your kidneys.

By now, you're well aware of how what you eat affects how you feel and your overall health. Everything you put in your mouth has a direct impact on your health and, for our purposes, your kidney health.

The basic principles of staying healthy are the following: maintaining a healthy weight, enjoying moderate exercise, getting enough sleep, not letting stress get to you. However, it is most important to keep an eye on what you eat and drink. This is true for everyone, but especially important for people who are watching out for their kidney health. Your diet can help you whether you are in prevention mode, trying to mitigate damage, or trying to prevent further damage from occurring. Conversely, your diet can harm you and cause further damage to your kidneys, revving up the speed of damage.

# Sodium

Sodium, or salt, is found in most processed foods, or added to flavor dishes. The problem with salt is that it can make your kidneys work harder, leading to damage and disease progression. It's easy to limit your salt levels, though, thanks to delicious aromatic veggies, herbs, and spices. You'll learn what to purchase in Stocking the Pantry (page 109) and in the Recipes chapter. Be mindful of processed foods that claim to be "low" or "reduced" sodium, as they may be higher in potassium, which can also damage your kidneys. Examples of high-salt foods include chips, canned soup, lunch meats, and most foods in cans or boxes.

Sodium is one of the body's major electrolytes, along with potassium and chloride. Electrolytes are important as they control the fluids going in and out of tissues and cells. (Sodium is also known as a mineral.) Because of this, sodium regulates blood pressure and blood volume. This is why when one eats a diet high in sodium, it can lead to high blood pressure. Also, sodium transmits impulses for nerve function and muscle contraction and aids in regulating the acid-base balance in the body.

Sodium is very prevalent in the food supply, and with CKD stages 1 through 4, controlling your intake of it is very important. While sodium plays a role in several functions of the body, those with kidney disease cannot eliminate excess fluid and sodium due to the kidneys not functioning properly. This is why too much sodium can be harmful—sodium and fluid can build up in your tissues and bloodstream, just as potassium and phosphorous can, and blood pressure increases. For those in stage 5 of CKD who require dialysis, your doctor and dietitian will require you to follow a low-sodium diet to control blood pressure and fluids. Monitoring your sodium intake will avoid blood pressure drops during dialysis and cramping.

Too much sodium in your diet may make it harder to control blood pressure. In stages 3 and 4 of CKD, excess sodium intake can increase your thirst level and make your body retain fluid. Fluid retention, also referred to as edema, makes your ankles, feet, face, and other body parts swell, and can be dangerous for your heart and lungs. Excess fluid in the bloodstream may make your heart work harder, enlarge it, and weaken it, and can even lead to heart failure. Sodium affects the lungs because fluid can build up, making it difficult to breathe and causing shortness of breath.

High blood pressure, or hypertension, is often called the "silent killer" because no known signs and symptoms are associated with it. Having your blood pressure monitored is important because hypertension can cause further damage to kidneys that are already unhealthy or have reduced function. This, as you may have guessed, can result in even more fluid, minerals, and waste building up in the body.

Lowering your sodium intake does not mean you have to cut out all the foods you love. You will find delicious replacements and experiment with new foods! Your taste buds will adjust, even if at first they're not so happy with it. Refer to the chart below to learn how to swap high-sodium foods for lower-sodium alternatives.

## HIGH-SODIUM FOOD SWAP-OUTS

| High-Sodium Foods | Lower-Sodium Alternatives |
| --- | --- |
| Canned vegetables | Use fresh or frozen vegetables (check the ingredients list to ensure there's no added salt, and always buy plain frozen vegetables that are not sauce-based). |
| Pasta sauce | Make your own by using a blender to combine tomatoes, onions, garlic, basil, oregano, black pepper, and olive oil. Add Mrs. Dash salt-free seasoning if desired. |
| Flavored instant oatmeal | Choose plain oats and add cinnamon and sliced fruit. |

## HIGH-SODIUM FOOD SWAP-OUTS

| High-Sodium Foods | Lower-Sodium Alternatives |
|---|---|
| Frozen chicken breast or rotisserie chicken | Purchase fresh chicken breast. |
| Microwave popcorn | Select air-popped popcorn or low-sodium rice cake snacks. |
| Luncheon meat | Buy store-roasted chicken, turkey, or roast beef (ask if it is made with salt or roast it yourself). |
| Canned soup | Always purchase low-sodium options, or make your own soup in a pot or slow cooker. |
| Cow's milk/dairy | Choose low-sodium coconut milk or make your own cashew milk; small amounts of natural cheese, such as blocks of cheese, are lower in sodium. |
| High-sodium sauces (barbecue sauce, soy sauce) | Substitute with low-sodium sauces, vinegar, or mustard. |
| Cured foods such as ham, bacon, or pork | Choose fresh beef, veal, pork, poultry, and fish. |

Remember, adjusting to these changes will not happen overnight. It will take days, weeks, or even months. Sooner than you know, low-sodium eating will be part of your daily routine and you won't have to *think* about doing it—you'll just do it.

# Potassium

Potassium, like salt, is a mineral found in many foods. Your body requires a balance of salt and potassium to work, but too much of either is dangerous and can lead to damage to your kidneys and other organs. Speak with your dietitian or health care practitioner about your specific recommended potassium intake. Foods high in potassium include oranges, raisins, spinach, beans, and brown rice. Foods lower in potassium (but still be mindful of levels) include apples, strawberries, lettuce, chicken, and white rice.

Potassium controls nerve and muscle function. For example, the heart beats at a normal rhythm because of potassium. High potassium levels can cause the heart to stop working. Low levels can cause muscle weakness and atrial fibrillation (also known as a-fib), which is an irregular, often rapid heart rate that can cause poor blood flow. Also, potassium aids in maintaining fluid and electrolyte balance, as well as pH level. Healthy kidneys help keep potassium within a normal level. As you have learned, when kidneys aren't functioning properly, these levels do not stay within the desired range and the level builds up in the body.

Hyperkalemia is the medical term that describes a high blood potassium level. In stage 5 CKD, also referred to as end stage renal disease (ESRD), dialysis is needed to regulate potassium. In CKD stages 1 through 4, there is usually no restriction in potassium unless blood work indicates that blood levels are high. When going through dialysis treatment, high-potassium foods must be limited because potassium levels can rise in between treatments. Refer to the chart below to learn how to swap high-potassium foods for lower-potassium alternatives.

For a list of high-, medium-, and low-potassium foods based on serving size, see Potassium Levels of Selected Foods on page 168.

## HIGH-POTASSIUM FOOD SWAP-OUTS

| High-Potassium Foods | Lower-Potassium Alternatives |
| --- | --- |
| Bananas, oranges, kiwi | Apples, berries, grapes |
| Cantaloupe or honeydew | Watermelon |
| Nectarines, mangos, papaya | Peaches, plums, or pineapple |
| Raisins and other dried fruit | Cranberries |
| Orange and prune juice | Apple, cranberry, or grape juice |
| Dried beans, peas | Green beans, wax beans, or snow peas |

## HIGH-POTASSIUM FOOD SWAP-OUTS

| High-Potassium Foods | Lower-Potassium Alternatives |
| --- | --- |
| Baked potatoes, french fries | Mashed potatoes, cauliflower mashed potatoes |
| Winter squash (like acorn) | Summer squash (like crookneck or zucchini) |
| Spinach | Iceberg lettuce or mustard greens |
| Tomatoes, tomato sauce, chili sauce | Onion, bell peppers, mushrooms, eggplant, broccoli, or garlic |
| Cow's milk yogurt or pudding | nondairy products such as KiteHill almond milk yogurt or SoDelicious coconut milk |
| Ice cream, frozen yogurt | Sherbet, sorbet, nondairy desserts |
| Chocolate desserts | Vanilla- or lemon-flavored desserts |
| Nuts, seeds | Unsalted popcorn, pretzels, or rice cakes |
| Salt substitutes and seasonings with potassium | Mrs. Dash seasoning |

Here are some general tips on reducing potassium in your foods:

- Remove excess liquid from canned fruit and vegetables.

- Leach high-potassium vegetables to remove some potassium. For example, cut and peel potatoes, place in a pot of water, and bring to a boil. Drain (this removes excess potassium), add fresh water, bring to a boil again, and cook until potatoes are tender.

- Read labels on packaged foods and avoid potassium chloride.

- Avoid a lot of enriched foods, which are products that add vitamins and minerals back into foods after they were removed during processing. Enriched foods often contain potassium, such as dry cereals and beverages, so read the nutrition labels carefully.

# Phosphorus

You may not be as familiar with phosphorous, but like salt and potassium, it's naturally found in a lot of foods. High-phosphorous foods are typically protein foods such as meats, poultry, fish, nuts, beans, legumes, and dairy products. Other foods high in phosphorous include whole grains, oatmeal, seeds, and soda. Foods lower in phosphorous (but still be mindful of levels) include sourdough, white bread and other white/refined food products, and plain popcorn.

Phosphorous works to keep your bones healthy. When your kidneys are working, your body keeps the exact right amount of phosphorous for ultimate functioning. But when your kidneys aren't doing so well, it can build up in your blood.

You may need to eat fewer high-phosphorous foods if your blood has high levels of phosphorous. When you don't consume the recommended portion sizes, phosphorous can build up in your blood. When this happens, your blood vessels, organs, and tissues can harden. It may also cause your skin to itch, as the body tries to decrease the dangerous levels. Also, when phosphorous levels are high, calcium can be pulled from your bones. This can cause weak bones that can easily can fracture or beak. High blood levels of phosphorous may be an early sign that kidney failure is already affecting your bones.

Speak to your dietitian or healthcare practitioner about your phosphorous limits. If your blood phosphorous levels remain high after changing your diet, your doctor may prescribe you phosphate binders. They are a medication taken with meals and snacks that reduce the absorption of phosphate by binding to it. The good news is that phosphate binders work wonders and often allow for a much more liberal diet. Phosphorous levels often remain elevated for individuals who do not comply with the recommended use of phosphate binders. However, if you have low phosphorus phosphorous levels due to the phosphate binders, add one serving of a high-phosphorous food per day. You can also decrease phosphate binders as directed by your doctor.

Whole grains have always been limited on the renal diet. However, the guidelines are undergoing a current shift. This is because while the phosphorous content in whole grains may be high, the phosphorous is bound to phytate, which requires an enzyme called phytase to be released in order to break down and absorb the phosphorous. Phytase is contained in some whole grains, but the enzyme is decreased in milling, processing, and preparation. Since most of us consume processed whole grains, the bioavailability of phosphorous from whole grains is low and our body does not absorb most of it. The restriction on whole grains is much looser now and is being reconsidered altogether. If your dietitian or doctor confirms you can consume whole grains, your diet will then provide much more fiber and protein.

The best whole grain choices with lower potassium and phosphorous content include barley, buckwheat, bulgur, popcorn, and wild rice. Whole grains with higher potassium and phosphorous content include amaranth, brown rice, millet, oats, quinoa, sorghum, spelt, teff, triticale, and wheat berries. For a list of high-, medium-, and low-phosphorous foods based on serving size, see Phosphorus Levels of Selected Foods on page 175.

Nondairy milk and creamers, such as almond, rice, coconut, and soy, normally contain less than half the phosphorous of dairy products. This means you can enjoy more milk with your cereal. Products do vary, so be sure to compare the labels when food shopping and choose the one with the lowest amounts of the minerals you're restricting.

The tricky part is that phosphorous (and potassium!) was not required to be listed on a Nutrition Facts label before July 2018, although some products may have listed its percent daily value. However, potassium is now required to be listed on the Nutrition Facts label, as it's a nutrient many Americans are deficient in.

Many food products provide the %DV rather than the amount in milligrams. The percent daily values are based off the recommended daily allowances (RDA) for healthy adults. So, because you have kidney dysfunction, the %DV can give you an idea of how much phosphorous or potassium is in the food product. For example, when the label says potassium is 5% DV, this means the food product has 5% of the recommended allowances of potassium or phosphorous for a person without kidney disease. Cereals with added nuts or whole grains usually contain more phosphorus and therefore contain 10% or more of the DV. Be mindful that even if there is no %DV listed, the mineral can still be in your food.

Use the following guide when potassium or phosphorus is listed to get a rough idea of the amount in the food:

Low phosphorous: Less than 5% DV

Medium phosphorous: 5–15% DV

High phosphorous: Greater than 15% DV

## Read the Ingredients List

Manufacturers add phosphorous additives, or "phos" additives, in processed foods to thicken, improve taste, preserve, and prevent discoloration of foods. A helpful hint is to consume products that don't have variations of the word phosphate listed in the ingredients list, including "phos" variations like the following:

- Calcium phosphate

- Phosphoric acid

- Sodium aluminum phosphate, pyrophosphate, polyphosphates

- Calcium phosphate

- Disodium phosphate

- Phosphoric acid

- Monopotassium phosphate

- Sodium acid pyrophosphate

- Sodium tripolyphosphate

A product that contains one of the above ingredients means that it has a phosphate additive and in turn contains a higher percentage of phosphorous. Many times food companies and manufacturers will provide nutrient information upon request. Just be sure to specify exactly what you're looking for.

These foods tend to contain phosphate additives (pay attention to ingredients list):

- Baking powder
- Pancakes
- Waffles
- Biscuits
- Instant puddings/sauces
- Processed deli meats
- Sodas and other beverages

To avoid this issue, try to prepare more meals at home with fresh ingredients. Limiting fast foods and processed foods is a good way to avoid accidentally consuming a high-phosphorous meal. For example, many frozen chicken products contain 28% to 100% more phosphorous than fresh chicken!

## Phosphorous Substitutes

The following list provides low-phosphorous alternatives to the foods you love. However, always be sure to read labels of your specific food products.

### HIGH-PHOSPHOROUS FOOD SWAP-OUTS

| High-Phosphorous Foods | Lower Phosphorous Alternatives |
|---|---|
| Beverages: sodas and other dark-colored beverages; canned and bottled drinks with phosphate additives | Homemade iced tea; apple cider |
| Brown rice or whole-wheat pasta | Refined "white" carbs: white rice, white pasta, couscous. |
| Whole wheat bread | White bread |
| Cereals made from bran, oats, or whole wheat | Cereals made from rice, corn, or white food products |
| Processed cheeses and spreads (e.g., Kraft cheeses) | A small amount of Brie, Parmesan, or cream cheese |

## HIGH-PHOSPHOROUS FOOD SWAP-OUTS

| High-Phosphorous Foods | Lower Phosphorous Alternatives |
| --- | --- |
| Cow's milk | Dairy-free milks: rice, coconut, or almond |
| Ice cream | Sherbet, Italian ice, dairy-free ice cream (coconut or almond) |
| Soups made with high-phosphorous ingredients (milk, dried peas, beans, lentils) | Broth or water-based soups |
| Quick breads, biscuits, cornbread, muffins, pancakes, or waffles | White dinner rolls, bread, bagels, or English muffins |
| Processed meats, such as bologna, ham, and hot dogs; and meat, poultry, or seafood with "phos" in the ingredients | All-natural lean beef, pork, lamb, poultry, seafood, or other fish without "phos" in the ingredients |
| Nuts and seeds | Popcorn or pretzels |
| Peanut butter and other nut butters | Jam, jelly, or honey |
| Whole wheat spaghetti | Spaghetti squash |

# Fluids

Water, tea, coffee, milk, creamer, soft drinks, juice, ice pops, ice cream, ice, sherbet, soups, gelatin, alcohol, other beverages, and, of course, water, are considered fluids. Although fruits and vegetables contain water, as well as foods cooked in water, such as rice and pasta, they aren't usually counted as fluid unless an individual is very sensitive to liquids because of poor heart or lung function.

Fluid is essential for life, but if your kidneys are struggling, you may not need as much as you did before. Damaged kidneys don't eliminate water as effectively as healthy ones, and too much fluid in your body can be dangerous. Having too much water in your body is called fluid overload or hypervolemia. If your body retains fluid, your ankles and feet may swell. It can also build up in your lungs, causing shortness of breath, high blood pressure, and other complications.

Speak to your doctor or healthcare practitioner about your fluid intake. You may need to be mindful of foods like soup, ice cream, and some fruits and vegetables that have high water content.

# Macronutrients

Now that you've learned about nutrients and minerals that have a direct impact on your kidneys, we'll discuss the macronutrients, which play a role in overall health. The three macronutrients are protein, fat, and carbohydrates.

## Protein

Protein is a building block for many of your body's processes. It's vital in how you heal and rebuild. But a diet high in protein can be hard on your kidneys, causing more damage. Check in with your dietitian or healthcare practitioner and see how much protein you should be eating based on your individual needs. Examples of high-protein foods include red meat, chicken, fish, eggs, and cheese.

While protein is a necessary macronutrient, patients with CKD often have to limit their protein intake. When protein is ingested, protein waste products are created. Healthy kidneys have millions of nephrons that assist in filtering this waste to remove it as urine. Unhealthy kidneys can't remove protein waste and it builds up in the blood. Your recommended protein intake will be based on your kidney disease state, nutritional status, and body size.

If you are in stages 1,2, or 3 of CKD, your protein intake may be limited to 12% to 15% of your daily calorie intake. If you are in stage 4 of CKD, you may be advised to decrease your intake to 10% of your daily caloric intake.

Limiting protein from animals, such as meat, poultry, fish, eggs, and dairy will reduce how hard your kidneys have to work. When eating an animal protein, always choose fresh, minimally processed meat, poultry, and fish. In fact, replacing animal protein with plant protein, such as beans, legumes, nuts, and nut butters, may help further reduce how hard your kidneys have to work. Plant proteins are naturally lower in unhealthy fats and can improve blood sugar control. However, they may be higher in potassium and phosphorous.

One ounce of the following cooked meat, poultry, and fish has about 7 grams of protein: beef, fish, lamb, pork, poultry, shellfish, veal, and wild game. Shellfish may be higher in sodium than the other foods listed.

Meat alternatives, such as those in the chart below, also have about 7 grams of protein per serving. Remember, the nuts may be high in potassium and the cheese may be high in sodium. Plant proteins are easier for your kidneys to process and thus are good protein choices.

| Meat Alternatives | Serving Size |
| --- | --- |
| Cheese, hard/unprocessed | 1 ounce |
| Cottage cheese | ¼ cup |
| Egg | 1 large |
| Egg substitute | ¼ cup |
| Nuts/peanuts, unsalted | 1 ounce |
| Peanut butter, unsalted | 2 tablespoons |
| Tempeh | ¼ cup |
| Tofu, firm | ¼ cup |

One serving (⅓ cup) of legumes (beans, peas, and lentils) have about 6 grams of protein per serving, including the following when boiled: black beans, black-eyed peas, broad beans, cannellini beans, chickpeas (garbanzo beans), lentils, lupin beans, mung beans, red kidney beans, soybeans, winged beans, and yellow beans. Hummus may be high in sodium and soybeans may be high in potassium.

The following chart shows protein foods with higher amounts of sodium, calories, potassium, and phosphorous. Choose these foods less often. One serving size averages about 7 grams of protein and 200 milligrams of sodium or more.

| Protein Foods to Limit | Serving Size |
|---|---|
| Bacon | 4 slices |
| Breakfast sausage | 1 ½ patties or 3 links |
| Salted and canned tuna, salmon, or sardines | ¼ cup |
| Cheese, processed (Kraft singles) | 1 ounce |
| Canned, salt-cooked beans and legumes | ⅓ cup |
| Deli meats, roast beef, turkey, ham, pastrami, salami | 1 ounce |
| Bratwursts, or Polish sausages | 2 ounces |
| Ham | 1 ounce |
| Organ meats | 1 ounce |
| Vegetarian/vegan meat alternatives: vegetable/soy burgers, soy cheese, soy sausage and links, soy meat crumbles | 1–2 ounces |

Source: © 2018 Academy of Nutrition and Dietetics, Nutrition Care Manual®. Accessed July 10, 2017. Adapted and reprinted with permission.

# Carbohydrates

Carbohydrates have caught a bad rap in recent years, but not all carbs are created equal. Good carbs are the easiest kind of energy for your body to break down and use as fuel. Did you know that vegetables and fruits are carbs too? They're excellent carb choices because they're full of vitamins, minerals, and fiber. Other healthy carbs include some whole and unrefined grains. Some carbs, however, are high in minerals that you may be directed to limit, such as potassium and phosphorus. Talk to your dietitian or healthcare practitioner about the appropriate levels of these minerals that you specifically should consume. Examples of unhealthy carbs to limit include candy, cookies, soda, juices, and white (also referred to as refined) bread/flour, pastry, and pasta. However, if you are prescribed to lower phosphorous intake, you actually will need to consume white food products, as the phosphorous content is much lower compared to whole wheat food varieties.

## Fats

Real, quality fats to include in your diet are the following:

**Fish and seafood:** sardines, mackerel, herring, black cod, wild salmon, clams, oysters, mussels, shrimp, scallops, crab, calamari, and octopus. Consider wild-caught fish.

*Limit:* lobster, tuna, catfish, king mackerel, Chilean sea bass, and swordfish.

**Land animals:** lamb, beef, bison, venison, chicken, duck, turkey, and eggs. Grass-fed, organic, sustainably raised animal products are important to consider.

**Dairy and dairy substitutes:** heavy cream, grass-fed butter, ghee, and unsweetened nut and seed milks (almond, cashew, hemp, hazelnut, and coconut).

*Avoid:* soy milk.

**Nuts and seeds:** almonds, macadamias, walnuts, pecans, and Brazil nuts; hemp, chia, pumpkin, sesame, and flaxseeds. Nut and seed butters are excellent without added sugars or bad oils.

*Consume in moderation:* peanuts and peanut butter.

**Oils:** unrefined coconut oil, coconut butter, olive oil, medium-chain triglyceride (MCT) oil, flaxseed oil, avocado oil, walnut oil, pumpkin seed oil, pistachio oil, and hemp oil. And...avocados. Always eat avocados!

*Avoid:* Safflower, soybean, sunflower, corn, canola, cottonseed oils, and other vegetable oils; margarine. Note: only use olive oil to drizzle on ready-to-eat foods such as salad, pasta, or avocado.

Keep in mind, processed foods are usually created with damaging fats, such as trans fats. Man-made foods are usually inflammatory. Excellent books to help you better understand this concept in depth are *Eat Fat, Get Thin* by Dr. Mark Hyman and *Fat for Fuel* by Dr. Joseph Mercola.

# Fruits and Vegetables

One of the most important highlights of the DASH diet is to eat a colorful plate (real colors from real food, nothing artificial!). Include vegetables in every single meal and one serving of fruit at least twice per day. Veggie omelets for breakfast, low-sodium turkey and kale wraps for lunch, and grilled chicken with spinach and roasted red-skinned potatoes for dinner, anyone?

Aim to fill half of your plate with vegetables. Veggies are so versatile, meaning you can have a side salad filled with raw veggies at one meal, steamed broccoli in garlic and olive oil at the next meal, and sweet potatoes in another. Eat your veggies raw, steamed, roasted, boiled, sautéed, or any way you desire! It is good to eat a mixture of both cooked and raw veggies, because, well, life is about balance. There's science behind this. For example, when tomatoes are heated, the nutritional value is actually enhanced. This isn't usually the case with veggies; however, lycopene, a phytochemical that gives tomatoes their red color and has nutritional benefits, is multiplied when heated. The Italians had it right all along, tomatoes are to be cooked! Lycopene is a powerful antioxidant which fights off cancer cells and reduces the risk of heart disease.

## Phytochemicals

Phytochemicals are compounds produced by plants and commonly found in fruits and vegetables. Under the umbrella of phytochemicals are carotenoids, polyphenols, anthocyanins, isoflavones, resveratrol, and flavonoids. When you eat a colorful plate of food, you are reaping the benefits from each color (each color of the rainbow provides different nutritional benefits). If you are aware of phytochemicals and the benefits of each, you may feel more inclined to eat a variety of fruits and vegetables. Also, you'll have greater knowledge of why it is so important to fill at least half of your plate with them. Since fruits and veggies are so highly recommended to consume, it's only fair to explain why they're so beneficial.

## Carotenoids

Carotenoids are plant pigments that provide yellow, orange, and red coloring to fruits and veggies; for example, red peppers, papayas, carrots, watermelon, and yellow squash. Beta-carotene is a type of carotenoid that provides orange pigmentation in carrots, sweet potatoes, and pumpkins. One of the excellent benefits of beta-carotene is its conversion to vitamin A. Under the umbrella of carotenoids are also lutein, zeaxanthin, and lycopene.

Carotenoids are also beneficial because they are antioxidants. Antioxidants prevent and reduce risks of diseases, as they fight free radicals in the body that cause oxidative stress. Also, they improve eyesight and prevent oxidative damage from our frequent use of technology. Tablet, smartphone, and television use cause oxidative stress because short-wave blue lights are absorbed. Lutein and zeaxanthin act as internal sunglasses that filter the blue light waves and protect the eyes. Because so many of us nowadays are attached to our electronic devices at the hip, it's important to consume carotenoids!

## Polyphenols

Polyphenols are the largest group of phytochemicals. Under the umbrella of polyphenols are flavonoids (discussed on page 71) and lignans (discussed on page 71). Polyphenols are strong antioxidants and can be found in raw cacao, legumes, spices, and fruits and vegetables. Long-term consumption of diets rich in plant polyphenols significantly protects against the development and progression of chronic illnesses, such as cancer, diabetes, cardiovascular disease, osteoporosis, neurodegenerative diseases, and aging. Epidemiological evidence suggests that polyphenols also aid in preventing asthma symptoms and protecting against obstructive lung disease.

## Anthocyanins

Anthocyanins are responsible for the dark red, blue, and purple pigments found in fruits and vegetables, such as blueberries, cranberries, strawberries, raspberries, blackberries, cherries, eggplants, grapes, red cabbage, and red apples. Anthocyanins, like other phytochemicals, are strong antioxidants that protect the liver, improve vision, reduce blood pressure, and reduce the risk of other serious diseases.

## Isoflavones

Isoflavones, also referred to as phytoestrogens, are plant compounds that mimic human estrogen and should be avoided. Isoflavones are found in legumes, mainly soybeans. Try to avoid excessive amounts of tofu, miso, edamame, soy milk, soy cheese, and soy yogurt as much as possible. Despite health claims that soy lowers risk of heart disease, an article in *The Journal of Nutrition* states that existing data on these claims are inconsistent or have inadequate support. Studies document potential safety concerns on increased consumption of soy products because they can cause hormonal disruptions in both women and men, inhibiting thyroid function and increasing breast cancer risk. They can block the body's natural estrogen receptors by binding to them.

## Resveratrol

This may be a phytochemical you're familiar with. This particular phytochemical is the reason why red wine has healthy benefits. For example, the French have low rates of heart disease; some speculate this is influenced by a daily, moderate consumption of red wine. The amount of resveratrol varies by the brand and type of grape the wine was produced from. Now, this doesn't mean to drink multiple glasses of wine per day. Cheap wines have been reported to be contaminated with arsenic. If you find a quality wine, be sure to still consume it in moderation, as alcohol can disrupt your gut microbiome, disrupt hormones, and damage the liver.

Resveratrol is produced by plants to protect against harmful organisms and environmental issues (such as lack of water). Resveratrol offers a variety of benefits to humans, such as protecting the heart and providing antioxidants that defend against disease. It can be found in grapes, peanuts, pistachios, blueberries, cranberries, mulberries, and dark chocolate.

## Flavonoids

These have several subclasses, including anthocyanins (discussed in detail on page 69), flavonols, flavanones, and isoflavones. Flavonols, found in apples, apricots, beans, broccoli, cherry tomatoes, chives, cranberries, kale, leeks, pears, onions, red grapes, and cherries are most commonly consumed. Similarly named flavanols can be found in dark chocolate, and regular consumption is known to reduce the risk of cardiovascular disease and lower blood pressure.

## Lignans

Lignans, a type of polyphenol, are found in seeds (flax, pumpkin, sunflower, poppy, sesame), grains, legumes, fruits, and veggies. The richest dietary source of lignans are flaxseeds. When you crush, mill, or grind flax seeds, they are most bioavailable and absorbable by the body. Buy flaxseeds ground, or grind them yourself in a coffee grinder, and add them into smoothies, oats, or on top of any dish. You can even make a homemade flaxseed bread.

Lignans have the ability to block the effects of estrogen, which could reduce the risk of hormone-associated cancers such as breast, uterine, ovarian, and prostate. Also, lignans are known to lower the risk of heart disease.

As you can see, each phytochemical provides tons of benefits. This is why consuming a mainly plant-based diet with different colors of fruits, veggies, nuts, seeds, beans, and legumes is crucial to your overall health Again, aim to fill half your plate with veggies, and some fruit. Aim to eat at least five servings of fruits and veggies daily. Not only will you reap the benefits of phytochemicals, but you'll naturally increase your consumption of potassium, and limit your sodium and unhealthy fat intake.

Some plants benefit from the cooking process while others are best consumed raw for great nutritional content. Also, while raw food contains live enzymes, it can be hard to digest and absorb all the nutrients. On the other hand, veggies cooked for long periods of time in poor-quality oil (vegetable oils) at high heat aren't a healthy option. A healthy option is vegetable soups made from quality ingredients with little to no added salt, and simmered for a long duration, providing your body with a boost of nutrients and fiber.

# How to Enjoy More Fruits and Vegetables

Now that you understand the importance of consuming fruits and veggies, let's put this thought into action. Eating more fruits and vegetables is a great way to add low-calorie foods that are full of color, flavor, texture, and most importantly, vitamins and minerals to your meals. Try the following tips to enjoy more fruits and vegetables every day:

1. If you're going to eat pizza, get your veggies in too! Try adding broccoli, spinach, green peppers, tomatoes, mushrooms, or zucchini as your toppings.

2. Mix up a breakfast smoothie made with quality protein, half an avocado, milk of choice, greens such as arugula, a tablespoon of almond butter, and half a banana.

3. Make a veggie wrap with roasted vegetables and feta cheese rolled in a sprouted grain tortilla (I recommend the Ezekiel bread made by the Food for Life brand).

4. Try making your own crunchy snacks, such as kale chips, sweet potato fries, or roasted chickpeas. There are tons of fun recipes online and in the end of this book.

5. Grill colorful vegetable kabobs packed with tomatoes, green and red peppers, mushrooms, and onions.

6. Add color to your salads with baby carrots, grape tomatoes, red cabbage, pomegranate seeds, spinach leaves, and berries. Yes, fruit is wonderful over a bed of greens!

7. Keep cut-up vegetables handy for breakfast omelets, midafternoon snacks, side dishes, lunch box additions, or a quick nibble while waiting for dinner. As soon as you purchase your veggies, make your life easier by chopping them that day and storing them in

an airtight container. Ready-to-eat favorites: red, green, or yellow peppers, broccoli or cauliflower florets, carrots, celery sticks, cucumbers, snap peas, and whole radishes. Dip them in home-made guacamole or hummus!

8. Place colorful fruit where everyone can easily grab it for an easy, on-the-go snack. Keep a bowl of fresh, just-ripe whole fruit in the center of your kitchen or dining table.

9. Make your own fruit salad full of berries, watermelon, grapes, and more. Divide it into small Tupperware containers for an easy grab-and-go snack. Pair it with a healthy fat and protein, such as a piece of cheese or 1 to 2 tablespoons of nut butter, to help stabilize blood sugars.

10. Get saucy with fruit. Puree apples, berries, peaches, or pears in a blender for a thick, sweet sauce on grilled or broiled seafood or poultry.

11. Make an omelet for dinner! Turn any omelet into a hearty meal with broccoli, squash, carrots, peppers, tomatoes, or onions, and top it with quality cheese. By quality cheese, we mean anything but Kraft.

12. Top half a baked sweet potato with broccoli and quality cheese.

13. Heat a homemade or low-sodium cup of vegetable soup as a snack or with a sandwich for lunch.

14. Add grated, shredded, or chopped vegetables such as zucchini, spinach, and carrots to turkey meatloaf, mashed potatoes, pasta sauce, and rice dishes.

15. Swap out high-calorie pasta for zucchini noodles! Buy them in the store or make them yourself with a spiralizer. Top with garlic and olive oil or a homemade turkey meat sauce.

16. Make fruit your dessert: Defrost half a frozen banana. Mash it until pureed. Add chopped nuts, quality protein powder, and a few tablespoons of oats. Yum!

17. Stock your freezer with frozen vegetables to steam or stir-fry for a quick side dish. Top with delicious herbs and spices for extra antioxidants and flavor.

18. Make your main dish a salad of dark, leafy greens and other colorful vegetables. Add chickpeas or tempeh. Toss in a homemade dressing of herbs and spices, olive oil, and apple cider vinegar.

Kidney-friendly superfoods to help promote optimal kidney function:

- Apples (high fiber, antioxidants, and anti-inflammatory properties)
- Apple cider vinegar (prevents kidney stones)
- Cabbage (low in potassium and rich in vitamins C and K, fiber, and phytochemicals)
- Cauliflower (high in vitamin C, folate, and fiber)
- Cherries (rich in antioxidants and phytochemicals)
- Garlic (antioxidant and anti-inflammatory properties)
- Grapes (rich in antioxidants; the skin is rich in resveratrol)
- Kale (low in potassium, high in vitamins A and C, iron-rich)
- Lemon juice (helps reduce kidney stone formation)
- Onion (low in potassium and rich in antioxidants with antihistamine properties)
- Pumpkin seeds (rich in antioxidants and magnesium, which helps reduce kidney stone risk)
- Red bell peppers (low in potassium and rich in vitamins A, B6, folic acid, and fiber)
- Sweet potatoes (rich in beta-carotene, vitamins A and C, B6, potassium, and fiber)
- Watermelon (rich in water with diuretic properties; helps produce more urine to flush toxins out)

Kidney-friendly herbs to help promote optimal kidney function:

- Dandelion (natural diuretic that strengthens kidney and soothes urinary tract issues)

- Ginger (cleanses the blood and kidneys of toxins)
- Nettle (natural diuretic that purifies blood and treats urinary tract infections; high in iron)
- Turmeric (antiseptic and anti-inflammatory to treat kidney infections and inflammation)

# Dialysis Nutrition Therapy

For patients who are in stage 5, or end stage renal disease (ESRD), the kidneys are working at less than 10%. Dialysis is needed to do the work of the failing kidneys or until a kidney transplant is possible. If and when you receive dialysis, you should have your dietitian prepare a personalized meal plan for you. It will generally be high in protein and lower in sodium, potassium, phosphorous, and fluids. There are two different types of dialysis treatments: hemodialysis (HD), which can be in-center traditional, in-center nocturnal, or home based, and peritoneal dialysis (PD). Your recommended diet is partly determined by which dialysis treatment you choose.

## Hemodialysis (HD)

Hemodialysis is a treatment option where blood is removed from the body by a complex set of tubes. The blood runs through a filter called a dialyzer, is cleaned, and is returned back to the patient. The blood comes in contact with dialysate when passing through the filter. Dialysate is the cleansing fluid placed in the abdomen that pulls extra waste and fluid out of the blood. Usually patients receive this type of dialysis three times per week for four-hour sessions. Its downsides include the complex treatment structure requiring frequent dialysis visits from the patient. Patients must also maintain a catheter or fistula in the arm or groin so that high blood flow areas may be accessed to perform dialysis.

# Home Hemodialysis (HHD)

This treatment option is a less complex version of regular hemodialysis, especially because it can be performed in the comfort of the patient's home. The overall system is simplified with a smaller dialysis machine and simpler blood tubing and connections. Because of its simplicity, many patients are choosing this method to preserve their independence and have more free time. The duration of the session for each patient varies and can be tailored to the individual's needs. Typically, it's performed up to six days per week with each session ranging from three to six hours.

There are shorter versions called short daily hemodialysis (SDHD). The longer versions, nocturnal hemodialysis (NHD), are usually conducted overnight. As you can see, there's more flexibility with HHD in terms of the frequency, duration, and the individual lifestyle.

# Peritoneal Dialysis (PD)

With this treatment option, a tube is placed in the abdominal cavity of the patient and fluid is exchanged at regular intervals. It can be tailored to the patient's needs and lifestyle. For example, it can be performed overnight while the patient is sleeping, or during the daytime with four manual exchanges that take about 15 to 30 minutes. More often than not, this is coined as the simplest form of dialysis and having high flexibility. This is the treatment option that has fewer lifestyle interruptions and fewer time constraints.

It is agreed uniformly that no dialysis treatment type is superior to the other in terms of clinical outcome, mortality, or cardiovascular deaths. HHD and PD afford some greater liberty from dietary restrictions, and greater lifestyle freedom.

The Division of Nephrology, Hypertension, and Renal Transplantation provides a wonderful overview of the advantages and limitations in each treatment mode:

|  | Advantages | Limitations |
|---|---|---|
| Hemodialysis (HD) | • Dialysis done at clinic by dialysis technicians and nurses | • Rigid schedule, limited flexibility<br>• Time commitment: ~20 hours a week<br>• Time allotment: no flexibility, as per dialysis unit<br>• Needs prior authorization and arrangement for travel<br>• Cannot travel to region without dialysis clinic<br>• Significant fluctuation of symptoms<br>• Needs AVF creation and needle access<br>• Needs transportation arrangements |
| Home Hemodialysis | • Flexible lifestyle and independence<br>• Time allotment: at patient convenience<br>• 5–6 times a week, so less symptomatic fluctuations<br>• Much higher freedom in dietary and fluid intake<br>• May eliminate the need for blood pressure medication and some of the other medications<br>• Easy to travel with, pack and go | • Needs a caregiver at least for the duration of dialysis, 5–6 times a week<br>• Time commitment: based on therapy, up to 22 hours a week<br>• Needs weaving into lifestyle<br>• Needs storage space of around half a closet<br>• Needs arteriovenous fistula (AVF) creation and needle access |

|  | Advantages | Limitations |
|---|---|---|
| Peritoneal Dialysis | • Flexible lifestyle and independence<br>• Time commitment: usually less than 10 hours per week<br>• Time allotment: as per patient convenience<br>• No needles<br>• Simple techniques, easy learning<br>• Continuous therapy, minimal fluctuation of symptoms<br>• Once a month clinic, so no need to travel repeatedly<br>• Easy personal travel, pack bags and go<br>• Can use Automated Peritoneal Dialysis (APD); connect the machine at night and go to sleep | • Needs weaving into lifestyle<br>• Abdominal catheter<br>• Does have passive sugar intake, so need to watch for weight gain<br>• Needs storage space of around half a closet |

Source: Division of Nephrology, Hypertension, and Renal Transplantation, "Home Hemodialysis and Peritoneal Dialysis," University of Florida Health, December 2017, http://nephrology.medicine.ufl.edu/patient-care/renal-replacement-therpay/home-dialysis.

# Dietary Requirements During Dialysis

## Calories

For PD patients, some calories come from the dialysate solution in the form of dextrose (a sugar). Because it provides calories, PD patients may need fewer calories per day than HD patients. Also, they will need fewer carbs, because the solution provides carbs.

## Sodium

Sodium intake should be limited to 2,000 milligrams or less daily with both HD and PD. PD is performed daily and, thus, the sodium restriction may be liberalized. Speak to your doctor or dietitian about this.

## Potassium

If you do PD, your potassium goal may be 3,000 to 4,000 milligrams per day. The recommendation for people on HD is usually 2,000 milligrams per day. PD is higher because potassium removal is more efficient, as treatments are daily.

## Calcium

Both treatments require a daily limit of 2,000 milligrams.

## Phosphorous

The recommended phosphorous limit is 800 to 1,000 milligrams per day for those on both HD and PD.

## Protein

Because dialysis is effective in removing protein waste from the blood, a low-protein diet is no longer necessary. Rather, because some amino acids (the building blocks of protein) are removed during dialysis, a higher protein intake is needed to replace the lost protein. PD can cause protein loss and HD can cause your body to break protein down faster than normal, which is why it's crucial to make an effort to get enough protein in. The protein requirements for both treatments are higher than CKD requirements. Be mindful that although you can increase your protein intake during dialysis, you still must reduce your intake of phosphorous. Many high-protein foods, such as milk, yogurt, cheese, dried beans, peas, lentils, nuts and seeds, peanut butter, and some soy products contain phosphorous or potassium.

A general guideline is to eat a high-protein food at each meal, or about 8 to 10 ounces of high-protein foods daily. Some protein powders are also safe for you to use. You can add these to foods like puddings, applesauce, shakes, fruit juice, low-sodium soups, or your milk of choice. You can always get unflavored protein powders that won't make your food taste like chocolate or vanilla.

## Fluid

Fluid restrictions usually take place when one begins dialysis, especially if it only occurs three days a week and if urine production is decreased.

If fluid limits are exceeded, extra water must be removed and negative side effects, such as the following, could occur: muscle cramping, low blood pressure, nausea, weakness, dizziness, and potentially, additional dialysis sessions to remove the fluid. Fluid restrictions go hand in hand with salt restriction. It can be easier to comply with fluid restrictions when sodium intake is well controlled.

Limiting how much sodium and fluid you have between dialysis treatments helps your body maintain the right amount of fluid, thus making it easier for your dialysis treatment to remove extra water. Sodium causes your body to hold on to water and increases your chance of fluid overload.

Fluid restrictions vary depending on an individual's needs. There are certain factors considered when determining the amount of fluid restriction, including the amount of weight gain between treatments, urine output, and swelling. A weight gain of more than 2.2 to 4.4 pounds between treatments is excessive. If one receives dialysis treatments frequently, such as five days per week, some restrictions are lifted because dialysate, the fluid that cleans the blood, takes care of extra sodium in the body.

Most people on PD have some kidney function left and, thus, still make some urine. Over time, this kidney function tends to decline. How much fluid you are allowed to have daily depends on how much urine you make.

Limiting fluids will make HD less daunting. HD patients tend to feel the negative effects of fluid imbalance, such as muscle cramps, more than PD patients. It's generally recommended that people on dialysis who do not make urine should have less than 4 cups, or 32 ounces, of fluid daily.

To avoid fluid overload, always track your fluid intake. Be aware that 30 milliliters is approximately 1 ounce. So, a 1,000-milliliter fluid restriction is about 33 ounces, which is a little over 4 cups. In most circumstances, dialysis patients need to limit their fluid intake to 32 ounces daily. You can purchase a container to mark up or keep a fluid journal. Also, it's important to manage your thirst so you don't mindlessly drink a glass of water. Use hard candies, ice chips, or frozen grapes when thirsty.

*Chapter 5*

# TIPS FOR SUCCESS ON THE DASH DIET

Changing your eating habits isn't always simple or desirable—but it's almost always necessary. Our food supply, food systems, and unlimited access to processed, high-sodium, high-sugar foods can make it very difficult to comply with a healthy eating regimen. However, you're here, reading this book, bettering yourself and your health. You have already taken the first step, the hardest step, which is why we know you can do this.

Right now, you can stop feeling bad about your eating habits, and learn how to slowly change your habits until they become a lifestyle. In this chapter, we'll discuss not only why falling off track a few times is okay (we're only human), but how to learn from it. We'll provide you with tips such as mindful eating, how to use spices and herbs to flavor food instead of salt, and how to make healthy meal swap-outs. Creating a new lifestyle for yourself will not happen overnight; it's a learning process that will take time, but the healthy habits you develop will last you a lifetime. That way, you never have to feel like you're dieting.

## Start with Small Changes

Starting with small changes that will become a part of your lifestyle will help with long-term weight loss and health. Small changes, such as eating a 4- to 6-ounce steak rather than a 12-ounce one, go a long way. Or, instead of having 5 ounces of chicken stir-fry, have 2 ounces of chicken and add in 3 ounces of lentils. Behaviors such as swapping a chocolate bar for a Greek yogurt with raw cacao powder or cacao nibs mixed in are more beneficial than you may think.

# Watch Your Portions

Choosing foods that are healthy and good for your kidneys is a great start, but eating too much of anything, even very healthy foods, can lead to problems. One way to keep track of your portions is by eating mindfully, as we'll discuss later in this chapter. You should always:

- Check the Nutrition Facts label and review the serving size. A lot of packaged foods contain more than one serving, but we tend to consume the entire package, because, well, it's one package. Make portion control easier: Remove the food from the package and separate it into individual servings so you know when to stop. It's always best to portion out the food right when you get home from the grocery store. This will set you up for success, especially for days that you're on the go.

- Always plan ahead. Plan your meals and snacks in advance, so you're not tempted by last-minute cravings or hungry in between meals. You can plan on Sundays, the night before, or on the morning of your busy day. Do what works best for you and your individual lifestyle. Remember that both consistency and getting into a realistic routine is key to sustainable, lifelong changes.

## Portion Distortion

If you're not familiar with food measurements, such as ounces or cups, then it's important to understand hand symbols that are equivalent to the measurements. Copy the chart on the next page onto a piece of paper or take a picture, and carry it with you (especially when dining out!). It's so easy to not be mindful or aware of portion sizes. Hopefully, using your hand will make understanding portion sizes easier.

| Hand Symbol | Equivalent | Foods |
|---|---|---|
| Make a fist | 1 cup (2 fists are 2 cups) | Rice, pasta, fruit |
| Your palm when you lay your hand out | 3 ounces | Meat, fish, poultry (it's okay to have up to 6 ounces of meat, which would be 2 palmfuls) |
| Your palm cupped | 1 ounce | Nuts, raisins |
| Thumb | 1 ounce/ 1 tablespoon | Peanut butter, hard cheese |
| Thumb tip | 1 teaspoon | Sugar (if you're going to have it) |
| Pointer finger | 1 ½ ounces | String cheese |

# Limit Meat

Treat meat as one part of the whole meal, rather than the focus. The best recommendation we have is to always plate your food as such: half veggies, a quarter protein or meat, and a quarter starch. Then, be sure to include some healthy fats, whether that is drizzling olive oil on veggies or adding half an avocado to your meals. Fruit is usually great to include at snacks. Always pair it with a healthy fat or protein source. For example, an apple with 2 tablespoons of nut butter or blueberries with string cheese.

As a general guideline, limit meat to less than 4 to 6 ounces per meal. If you're used to eating large portions of meat, cut them by a third every few weeks. Including more plant-based meals, such as a quinoa and fresh beans with sautéed vegetables, is a great way to naturally lower sodium content and decrease excess meat intake. You may also be interested in doing Meatless Mondays where you only consume plant-based meals! Also, if you have meat for lunch, you typically don't need it for dinner, as long as you're getting your protein from a nonmeat source, such as lentils or tempeh.

## Keep Snacks Simple and Balanced

Snack choices should have very short ingredients lists and should be made of real and whole foods. They should be a nice balance of protein, fat, and carbs and should be limited in excess calories, sodium, trans fats, and sugar. When snacking, keep in mind it should always be a combination of at least two of the following: protein, fat, and carbs. A single portion should follow these guidelines:

- **Protein:** about half of the palm of your hand. For meals, your full palm.
- **Fat:** at least 2 tablespoons every time you eat (avocados, coconut oil, nuts/seeds, nut butter, etc.).
- **Starchy carbs:** ½ cup (corn, peas, beets, squash, yams, sweet potatoes, plantains). They are denser and increase blood sugar more quickly than non-starchy vegetables.
- **Non-starchy carbs:** Unlimited! They have such little effect on blood sugar levels and are full of vitamins, minerals, and fiber. Foods in this category include broccoli, cauliflower, spinach, carrots, cabbage, kale, peppers, green beans, cucumbers, and asparagus.

# Set SMART Goals

In this day and age, we have become accustomed to instant results. Why? Because look at how our lifestyles have evolved from previous times. You can receive mail in the blink of a second rather than waiting for it come via snail mail. You can deposit checks on your cell phone rather than driving to the bank. What's more, you can get same-day delivery service for groceries.

When it comes to nutrition, setting goals is one of the most important things you can do to achieve a new, healthy lifestyle. But you must understand that change and achieving goals takes more than thoughts and a few seconds to accomplish. It takes time, dedication, and most importantly, patience. Have a plan of action and set goals with a focus on where you want your body and health to be is crucial. Many times we focus on the end goal but forget to plan for the game and how we'll achieve it. Without a plan of action, the events in between can get messy and control lost. You can plan your meals with the chart on page 182 to help make following the DASH diet easier.

SMART goal setting can bring structure to your goals and plan. It allows you to track your progress and keep you on track. Additionally, it allows you to have that set plan of action which allows you to turn your goals into realities. The acronym SMART stands for the following:

Specific

Measurable

Attainable

Realistic

Timely

When setting up your goals, ask yourself the follow questions:

• What exactly do I want to achieve?

• Why do I want to achieve them?

• Where? When? How? With Whom?

• What are some issues I may encounter along the way?

• How will I surpass a roadblock?

For example, rather than making a goal of "I will get more exercise on the weekend," be as specific as this: "I will run for 20 minutes both Saturday and Sunday at 9:00 a.m." Here are some additional tips:

- Start small. This is called short-term goal setting. Think about what you can realistically accomplish over the next few weeks. Don't make the goal list too long; perhaps set a maximum of four goals for two to three weeks.

- Write the goals down. Have them in a common view, such as on the fridge or on your desk. Writing goals down shows you are committed and focused. Having the goals in front of you often will give you accountability.

- After two to three weeks, sit down and reflect on your goals. Did you meet them? If not, why? Did you set unrealistic goals and expectations for yourself?

- Celebrate small successes. Achieving even one goal can boost your confidence and motivation. And always remember, small achievements lead to a great, large success.

- Don't use the words "never" or "always." For example, don't say "I will never eat French fries again." The all-or-nothing attitude sets you up for failure and often sends you back to poor habits. Again, you must consider if your goal is realistic or not. It's unrealistic to give up a common food forever. And, remember, there are always healthy alternatives and substitutions for your favorite foods. A better, realistic goal would be "I will substitute French fries for homemade, hand-cut sweet potato wedges when I am craving them."

- Lastly, never expect perfection. Failure will happen and you may disappoint yourself. Never give up when this happens. Use failure as a reason to understand what went wrong. Patience and perseverance are keys to long-term success.

I hope you have been convinced not to give up, to keep pushing, and to be in control of your health once and for all. The power of your health lies in your hands. So, go on, right now, make a goal for the next few weeks. Even if the goal is to read one more chapter in this book or to test a recipe.

# Eat Mindfully

You may have heard about the concept of mindfulness before. It's become a popular wellness practice in the past several years as a way to reduce stress, relieve anxiety, and yes, even to eat better. Mindfulness is simply the concept of being present in the moment. It's not religious, and you don't need to ascribe to any particular morals or values. All you need to do is slow down. Focus your attention on what you're doing in the present moment; not what you're going to do later, not what you did today or five years ago, not even what is on the television.

You're going to focus on the sensory experience that is happening *right now*. Wild, right?

Mindful eating is trying to be aware of all of the sensations and feelings that come with eating: what you are tasting, smelling, feeling, hearing, touching, seeing. How do these things make you feel about your food choice? Do you feel nourished? Do you feel full? When you eat mindfully, you may chew more slowly and be less likely to eat empty calories that don't have a lot of nutritional value.

But, as it does, life can get in the way of our good intentions to eat every bite mindfully. With families, jobs, and a million other distractions, we may find ourselves more distracted from mindfulness than we like.

Mindful eating is one of the best ways to be in tune with your body and be present in the moment of eating. It is a tool used by many health professionals to improve eating behaviors, encourage weight control, and foster a healthy relationship with food. How often do you sit in front of the TV, thoughtlessly eating chips? Before you know it, the whole bag is gone. Or how often have you eaten over the stove, standing up? How often have you eaten so fast that you haven't even enjoyed the taste of the food or listened to hunger cues?

We often don't make time for meals, nor do we savor our food. We rarely sit down to eat as a family. We don't listen to hunger cues or satiety cues (fullness cues).

The following are the principles of mindful eating as per the Center for Mindful Eating:

### Principles of Mindfulness:

1. Mindfulness is paying attention, deliberately and without judgment.

2. Mindfulness encompasses both internal processes and external environments.

3. Mindfulness is being aware of what is present for you mentally, emotionally, and physically in each moment.

4. With practice, mindfulness cultivates the possibility of freeing yourself of reactive, habitual patterns of thinking, feeling, and acting.

5. Mindfulness promotes balance, choice, wisdom, and acceptance of what is.

### Mindful Eating Is:

1. Allowing yourself to become aware of the positive and nurturing opportunities that are available through food preparation and consumption by respecting your own inner wisdom.

2. Choosing to eat food that is both pleasing to you and nourishing to your body by using all your senses to explore, savor, and taste.

3. Acknowledging responses to food (likes, neutral, or dislikes) without judgment.

4. Learning to be aware of physical hunger and satiety cues to guide your decision to begin eating and to stop eating.

### Someone Who Eats Mindfully:

1. Acknowledges that there is no right or wrong way to eat, but varying degrees of awareness surrounding the experience of food.

2. Accepts that their eating experiences are unique.

3. Is an individual who, by choice, directs their awareness to all aspects of food and eating on a moment-by-moment basis.

4. Looks at the immediate choices and direct experiences associated with food and eating, not to the distant health outcomes of those choices.

5. Is aware of and reflects on the effects caused by unmindful eating.

6. Experiences insight about how they can act to achieve specific health goals as they become more attuned to the direct experience of eating and feelings of health.

7. Becomes aware of the interconnection of earth, living beings, and cultural practices and the impact their food choices have on those systems.

## Be Aware

Mindful eating includes being aware of all that food has to offer, including how it's prepared and the act of consuming it. Foods can be nutritious yet enjoyable, and mindful eaters acknowledge food preferences without judgment, choosing which food to eat through knowledge. This means, instead of getting angry that French fries are your favorite food, acknowledging it. Understanding that it's okay French fries are your favorite food, but having the knowledge that you can't eat them every day, is a part of mindful eating. Cooking or purchasing healthier but delicious alternatives to French fries, such as homemade baked sweet potato fries, is part of mindful eating. The very act of eating when hungry, rather than eating due to seeing or smelling somebody else consume a cheeseburger, is mindful eating. Megrette Fletcher, MEd, RD, CDE, cofounder of the Center for Mindful Eating, states, "Either you're really physically hungry or there's another trigger for eating." Mindful awareness allows you to notice your state of mind and current experience.

Mindful eating takes practice and certainly doesn't occur overnight. People tend to overeat due to poor habits and unconscious behaviors that have been repeated for years. Some people are not even *aware* of their poor habits. Once there's awareness, action can be taken. The concept includes making adjustments in life that will avoid triggers that may force individuals to consume too much food or make poor food choices.

The following strategies work wonders:

- Eat on smaller plates.

- Pay attention to serving sizes.

- Drink from smaller cups.

- Portion food into containers.

- Don't purchase unhealthy foods at the grocery store to avoid seeing them in the cabinet.

- Share a dinner plate at restaurants.

- Don't even glance at the dessert menu.

- Make a meal schedule for the week to stay on track.

- Take a different route to work to avoid stopping at the fast-food restaurant.

There are a few steps to be taken to facilitate behavior change. Check the boxes after you've answered each question for yourself.

❑ Why do I eat? (Hunger, boredom, fell victim to advertisements, somebody told me to, etc.)

❑ When do I want to eat? (When the clock hits a certain time, in the morning when I'm super hungry, at night because it's habit, or when I'm feeling emotional)

❑ What do I eat? (Convenience food, food that tastes good, food that's nutritious, food that'll make me lean, comfort food, food I've eaten my whole life)

❑ How do I eat? (Rushed, mindfully, distracted, secretive, slowly)

❑ How much do I eat? (Until I feel full, until I feel sick, only the food on the plate that was portioned out perfectly, five times more than the recommended serving size, the same amount as usual due to habit)

❑ Where does the energy go? (Causes guilt and shame, causes the feeling of strength, causes lethargy)

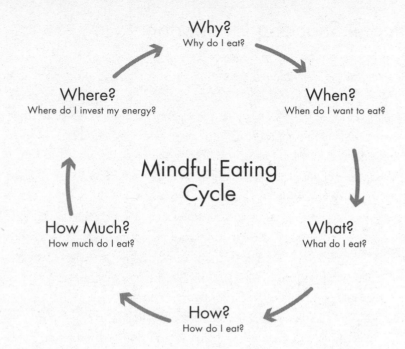

Why?
Why do I eat?

Where?
Where do I invest my energy?

When?
When do I want to eat?

Mindful Eating Cycle

How Much?
How much do I eat?

What?
What do I eat?

How?
How do I eat?

Mindful eating cycle graphic from *Eat What You Love, Love What You Eat* by Michelle May.

You may never have asked yourself these questions before. In our technological, on-the-go society, it's rare to take this sort of time. The first time around, you may not be honest with yourself—that's normal. Continue to ask yourself these questions daily. This will boost your awareness of what you're eating, why you're eating, and how often you're eating. Moreover, this very act can aid you in ditching poor nutritional and behavioral habits. You have the ability to change old behaviors into positive ones. However, be aware that this technique should only provide insight to your eating habits. Do not judge your habits. There is no right or wrong answer. For example, if your answer to "How do I eat?" was "rushed," do not get angry or emotional about this or demand yourself to change this behavior immediately. Instead, use this understanding and awareness to brainstorm how you can make a more informed choice next time. Just as poor habits took years to develop, it can take some time to break out of them.

# Mindful Snacking Is Important

Do not underestimate the importance of snacking. Snacking helps keep you energized in between meals and prevents you from overeating during mealtime. However, there's a difference between snacking and grazing. Snacking is done at a set time, provides good nutrition, is portioned out, and is eaten for the right reason. Grazing is snacking mindlessly without paying attention to the portion or, simply snacking out of boredom.

Many people snack to alleviate the feeling of boredom or out of habit (for example, when watching your favorite TV show) but it's important to listen to your stomach rather than your mind. If you're not actually hungry, try to find another activity to do to cure your boredom, such as reading a book, going for a walk, or cleaning up. Drink a glass of water when you think you're hungry to make sure you are hungry and not thirsty. Snacking is also tempting due to constant food advertisements for chips, candy, and other processed foods. Don't give in to the temptations!

Certain events, such as parties or going to the movie theater, might cause you to snack even if you're not hungry. Always eat a meal beforehand so you're not going into a place like this hungry or, better yet, bring your own snacks with you! Also, try to be mindful of portion sizes when you occasionally snack on unhealthier food choices. You won't feel as bad if you eat a portion of chips, or two cookies, rather than the whole bag or box.

Snacking is so important because it supports your metabolism and keeps your blood sugar levels balanced (which keeps cravings away, stabilizes mood, and keeps energy levels up!). Snacking on healthy foods can also help keep your mind alert—nobody can focus when they're hungry! Snacking provides your body with nutrients and can prevent sleepiness and grumpiness. When you don't snack and wait long periods in between meals, your body learns to live in "starvation mode," which makes your metabolism plummet. Your body then hangs onto extra energy at meals by turning it into fat, because it's expecting it'll need that fat for energy in case you don't eat again.

# How Does This Relate to You?

Mindfulness-Based Eating Awareness Training is a program developed by Jean Kristeller, PhD, who combines mindful eating experiences, meditation, and discussion on how awareness can help inform participants about their behaviors and experiences surrounding food. This program was used in a randomized, prospective, controlled study published in the *Journal of the Academy of Nutrition and Dietetics*. It encouraged participants to combine inner wisdom (an awareness of food) and outer wisdom (a knowledge about the concerns of diabetes and nutrition). The first group practiced mindful eating exercises, meditation, and basic information regarding diabetes and nutrition. The second group received intense counseling sessions on managing diabetes, calorie needs and goals, and exercise requirements. Both groups experienced significant weight loss, improved blood sugar levels, increased fiber intake, and lower trans fat and sugar consumption. Because there were no significant differences in weight or blood sugar control between the two groups, mindful eating can be considered effective for diabetes patients.

The same concept can be applied to you, whether you have high blood pressure, kidney failure, or another nutrition-related disease. While it's important to understand your nutritional needs and the concerns of your disease state, it's equally important to be aware overall of what you are putting in your body, when, and why. Thus, research has been done behind the concept of mindful eating and has proven it to be effective and work for people, whether they have a disease such as diabetes or they're obese and cannot control their eating habits.

# Mindful Eating Exercises

- Create a hunger scale ranging from 0 to 10 (0 being the least hungry and 10 being the most hungry).
- What does a 0 feel like? (Nausea, fullness, bloating, tired, guilt, or another emotion, such as sadness)

- What does a 10 feel like? (Shakiness, headaches, irritability, sleepiness)
- Where are you right now on the hunger scale? (0 to 10)
- What do you notice about your body that made you choose that particular number?

Now, keep a journal of your hunger rating before, during, and after each meal for three days. Pay close attention to physical cues (stomach growling, feeling of fullness, bloating, etc.) that led to your choice. This will help you understand physical cues from your body that will get you better adapted to mindful eating.

## Food Experiment

- Hold a small piece of food in your hand, such as a raisin, grape, piece of cheese, or a piece of chocolate.
- Observe the appearance, texture, and aroma.
- Do you notice any changes in your body while you observe this food? (salivation, impatience, anticipation, or nothing)
- Place the food in your mouth, but do not chew it. Wait 30 seconds and then chew.
- What did you notice about the flavor or texture before you began chewing the food? What about after you started chewing?
- How does this experience compare with your typical experience with eating?

You may realize that you never observe food, feel the texture in your mouth, or savor it. You may understand that you've been mindlessly consuming food, putting it in your mouth and rapidly devouring it. With your newfound knowledge of mindful eating, rest assured you'll be eating more slowly, choosing when to eat based on your body's needs rather than your mind's desires, and choosing foods to fuel your body rather than falling victim to food advertisements.

Here are some ways you can incorporate mindful eating into your every day:

## 1. Slow Down

Did you know that your body is actually satiated, or full, about 20 minutes before your brain clues you in? That's a long lag time and a big opportunity to overeat, especially if you're eating quickly and mindlessly.

But if you slow down, you can give your body and brain a chance to transmit and receive the signals at the right moment. Try to sit down when you eat instead of standing, or worse, driving. Try to chew thoroughly. Set your utensils down between bites.

## 2. Check In

Sometimes we eat because we're truly hungry, but sometimes we eat because we're supposed to eat, or scheduled to eat, or because we're bored, upset, or anxious (or a million other emotional triggers). Use your mind to check in with your body: Are you hungry or not? Is your stomach growling? Does your energy feel low? Those are signals to eat. Two tips to combat boredom eating are 1) Drink a glass of water. If you're still craving something half an hour later, then go ahead and eat it, and 2) Are you hungry enough to eat an apple or a cup of carrots? If you're truly hungry, it won't be for something specific—like a donut.

## 3. Plan Ahead

Think of the last time you made a not-so-great food choice. What was it? Why was it? Was it something sweet, salty, or high in fat? Were you bored, stressed, or lonely? Was it a snap decision?

Clear out your cabinets of anything you might turn to out of habit or in times of stress. Replace them with healthy snacks. Plan meals that are nutritious and filling so you'll be less tempted to snack.

# DASH Side Effects

There are two types of fiber: soluble and insoluble. Fiber is found in plant foods, and almost every plant contains both types. Because DASH is high in fruits, vegetables, and whole grain foods, you may experience some bloating and diarrhea from all the fiber you're consuming.

Insoluble fiber, such as the fiber in wheat, does not dissolve in water and is not acted on by colon bacteria; therefore, it does not create gassiness. Insoluble fiber is important because it binds to the water within the colon, promoting a large, bulky stool. Ultimately, this improves regularity with going to the bathroom. Going to the bathroom on a regular basis is a sign of good health and diet! There is an inverse association between insoluble fiber intake and blood pressure, total cholesterol levels, and triglycerides. This means the more insoluble fiber you consume, the less likely you are to develop these diseases. Fiber lowers LDL cholesterol by interfering with the absorption of cholesterol. Think about the Mediterranean diet, a high-fiber diet full of fruits, vegetables, beans, and whole grains. The heart disease risk for those on this diet is much lower than those who consume typical foods in the SAD.

Prebiotic fibers are a special type of soluble fiber that are underappreciated. There's much talk about probiotics, but not as much about prebiotics, which are the food for probiotics. When soluble fiber is broken down, prebiotics are released. Some prebiotics you may have heard of are inulin and oligofructose. They have significant health benefits, such as improving regularity, since the human body cannot break them down. Once prebiotics pass through the small intestine, they reach the colon and are fermented by gut microflora, or bacteria.

Since prebiotics become fuel for the good bacteria that live in your gut, they work with probiotics to maintain balance and diversity of good intestinal bacteria. Prebiotic food sources include under-ripe bananas, raw garlic, raw or cooked onions, raw leeks, raw chicory root, raw Jerusalem artichokes, and raw dandelion greens. This is another example of why it's good to include raw veggies in your diet. When you cook these food sources, some of the precious prebiotic fiber is lost. Foods that contain both prebiotics and probiotics are fermented dairy products such as yogurt, cheese, kefir, and sour cream. Together, they have a symbiotic relationship. In this case, the definition of their symbiotic relationship is that they provide a beneficial balance that can only be achieved by working together.

Soluble fiber, such as the fiber in oats and beans, does dissolve in water and is fermented by colon bacteria. These bacteria are what create colon gas and feelings of bloating. The key with fiber is to get a good balance of its food sources, which is why eating a varied and balanced diet is important! If you are experiencing lots of gas and flatulence, cut back on soluble fiber foods first. When adding fiber, gradually increase your intake of it to reduce some of the side effects such as gas, cramps, and diarrhea. Add one high-fiber food, get your body adjusted to it, and then continue adding more. Eventually, aim to include fiber at every meal. Also, drinking plenty of water with fibrous foods helps to keep it moving through your digestive tract.

Fiber contributes to good health in plenty of ways. Not only does it keep food moving smoothly and regularly through your body, aiding in elimination, but it helps prevent heart disease, too. Due to fiber's structure and our inability to absorb it, it passes through the digestive system unabsorbed by digestive enzymes within the stomach. It removes toxins, waste, fat, and cholesterol particles from the gut. Thus, it contributes to digestion and detoxification. Additionally, it makes you feel full, which aids in weight loss as you're less likely to snack or continue eating when you're not hungry. Another great benefit of fiber is that it helps control blood sugar levels and prevent diabetes. This is because soluble fiber slows down digestion, which prevents spikes in blood sugar levels as the absorption of carbs is reduced.

Ideally, we should be getting more than 25 to 30 grams of fiber per day. Most of us only take in approximately 15 grams per day. Consuming a variety of fruits, veggies, beans, legumes, and whole grains can help you reach this. When looking at food labels, be sure to choose whole grain foods (such as breads, oats, barley) with at least 2 grams of fiber per serving. Consuming a variety of fibrous foods will allow you to get all the nutrients you need each day. Some high-fiber foods include split peas, lentils, black beans, mung beans, and figs. You can ensure you're getting fiber in when you eat the peels and skins of foods in fruits and vegetables, such as apples, cucumbers, and potatoes.

# Get to Know Your Nutrition Facts Label

The Nutrition Facts label is your guide to understanding what is inside processed and packaged food. Keep this excellent tool under your belt to help you choose the best foods and make informed decisions, especially in regard to your prescribed diet.

Listed on all packaged foods, the Nutrition Facts label is the best source of quick nutritional information. Fresh fruits and vegetables, meat, poultry, freshly baked goods, and seafood are not required to have one. To the right is a sample of the new Nutrition Facts label that will begin appearing in July 2018.

**Nutrition Facts**

8 servings per container
Serving size        2/3 cup (55g)

Amount per serving
Calories        **230**

| | % Daily Value* |
|---|---|
| **Total Fat** 8g | **10%** |
| Saturated Fat 1g | **5%** |
| Trans Fat 0g | |
| **Cholesterol** 0mg | **0%** |
| **Sodium** 160mg | **7%** |
| **Total Carbohydrate** 37g | **13%** |
| Dietary Fiber 4g | **14%** |
| Total Sugars 12g | |
| Includes 10g Added Sugars | **20%** |
| **Protein** 3g | |
| Vitamin D 2mcg | 10% |
| Calcium 260mg | 20% |
| Iron 8mg | 45% |
| Potassium 235mg | 6% |

* The % Daily Value (DV) tells you how much a nutrient in a serving of food contributes to a daily diet. 2,000 calories a day is used for general nutrition advice.

## Serving Size and Servings Per Container

All information listed on the label is based on the serving size. Many of us consume double or triple the recommended portion size. If you eat more than one serving, you'll be taking in more calories and nutrients than the amount listed on the label, and vice versa if you eat less than the serving size.

Here's an example of a food label of a bag of chips:

Serving size: 20 chips

Servings per container: 6

Calories: 100

It's common for people glance at the label, see that it says 100 calories, and then proceed to eat the entire bag of chips. But that 100 calories is for a sixth of the bag (because there are six servings), so really, 600 calories were consumed. This is why it's crucial to look at the serving size *and* how many servings per container there are. The servings per container does not jump out at you, which is why it's common to consume multiple servings. Paying attention to this can really prevent you from overeating and consuming more food than you need.

Comparing similar food products is usually simple because they likely have the same serving size. For example, one serving of salad dressing is always 2 tablespoons, regardless of the brand. This makes comparing the labels of different brands easy (no math involved!).

## % Daily Value

How can you tell if a food is high or low in a particular nutrient? Look at the %DV, located on the right side, as it shows if there's a small or large amount of a certain nutrient.

Five percent or less of the DV is low in a nutrient and 20% or more of the DV is high in a nutrient. This is beneficial when restricting sodium on the DASH diet, as you can see at a glance if the food is low or high in sodium.

## The Beloved Ingredients List

The ingredients list is crucial to look at and should be one of the main deciding factors when choosing a food product. The front of the package can tell you whatever it wants, but the ingredients list is where you'll see exactly what the food product is made up of. You'll see if the product is made up of wholesome, real food ingredients or if it's a highly processed food filled with additives and man-made chemicals (these usually consist of words you can't pronounce).

A super-long ingredients list with words you cannot pronounce indicates that the food is highly processed (and this is something you should stay away from!). Processed foods are almost always found in boxes, containers, plastic wrap, or cans. For example, cereal, canned soup, chips, cookies, microwaveable meals, and even drinks are highly processed.

## Carbohydrate Content

When looking at a food's carb content, what's most important is to see many grams of fiber are listed under the carbs on the Nutrition Facts label. To calculate the net carb count, simply subtract the number of grams of fiber from the total number of carb grams. The fiber does not impact blood sugar, so it doesn't "count," so to speak.

The new Nutrition Facts label also will have added sugars listed under fiber, so you will know if a food product has sugar added to it or if the sugar is naturally occurring, like in fruit. Stay away from added sugars as much as possible.

## Sodium Content

All Nutrition Facts labels have milligrams of sodium listed. Follow these steps when reading the sodium information on the label:

1. Know how much sodium you are allowed each day. Remember that there are 1,000 milligrams in 1 gram. If your diet prescription is 2 grams of sodium, that means you cannot consume more than 2,000 milligrams per day.

2. Look at the package label. Check the serving size. Try to eat a portion based on the serving size. Compare the sodium level to your daily allowance. If the sodium level is 500 milligrams or more per serving, the item is not a good choice, because that's a quarter of your daily sodium intake allowance.

3. Compare labels of similar products. Select the lowest sodium level for the same serving size.

# Avoid Processed Foods

Focus on purchasing real, fresh, whole foods such as fruits, veggies, meats, and cheeses. Shop the perimeter of the supermarket, where you can find most of these preferable foods. And, yes, your fresh food will expire MUCH more quickly than your processed foods, but a food shopping list with the right amount of foods needed for the week will prevent you from throwing out expired food. Also, you won't have high-sodium, high-sugar, highly preserved food sitting in your shelves, which means less temptation and better health outcomes.

You should be able to judge a food product in three steps.

1. **Look at the serving size.** What is the serving size and how many servings are in the product? Also, how many calories are in the serving you will be eating? Don't forget to look at the levels of sugar, trans fat, and sodium.

2. **Use the %DV on the right-hand side.** Is this a wise food choice? Will you be getting an abundance of good nutrients versus the bad ones? Remember, 5% or less of the DV is low, and 20% or more of the DV is high.

3. **Review the ingredients list.** How long is the ingredients list? Does it have words you can't recognize or pronounce?

Go to https://www.davita.com/diet-helper to help you with kidney-friendly meal planning. After creating an account, you can plan meals, track what you eat, create a grocery list, compare local food deals, navigate restaurant menus with kidney-friendly guides, track fluid intake, and much more! This website is a helpful tool to help manage your diet.

## Understand Industry Terms for Sodium

The front of a food product may make claims regarding sodium that you need to be aware of. Just because a product says it has reduced sodium does not mean it's a good choice for you. For example, if a food product originally had 1,200 milligrams of sodium and then reduced it by 25%, it still would not be a good choice.

- Sodium Free: Only a very small amount of sodium per serving.
- Very Low Sodium: 35 mg or less per serving.
- Low Sodium: 140 mg or less per serving.
- Reduced Sodium: Foods in which the level of sodium is reduced by 25%.
- Light or Lite in Sodium: Foods in which the sodium is reduced by at least 50%.

Helpful hint: If salt is listed in the first five ingredients, the item is probably too high in sodium to use. That's because the ingredients list goes in order of descending weight. So, if the first ingredient is sugar, the product's main and heaviest ingredient, by weight, is sugar.

# Dining Out

When you decide to commit to a new diet or nutrition plan, it can be difficult to know what you should eat and what you should avoid when you dine out. It can be overwhelming to have to make those choices without having any information beforehand. This can lead to falling off the wagon, so to speak, and making choices that you might regret later. The good news is that on the DASH diet, there are still a lot of foods you can enjoy. You don't need to be left out of the fun of dining out, and you can be empowered to make good, healthy, and delicious choices. In this section, we'll provide dining out tips, like what to look for in restaurant menus, what to avoid, what to ask for, and how to have conversations with your server or companions about your dietary needs. No one should make you feel bad about making positive choices for your health. We'll help you have those conversations.

We dine out far more often than our ancestors ever did. Restaurants, cafes, and coffee shops are all readily available. We're also living in the age of foodies who dine out to explore new food combinations (such as sushi burritos) and take food pictures specifically for Instagram likes. That being said, it's no wonder the incidence of hypertension has increased over the years.

Restaurant food is high in sodium despite restaurant claims such as ditching artificial ingredients or getting rid of genetically modified items. But, have you noticed there aren't too many restaurants claiming they've lowered their sodium content? Well, it's not easy for restaurants, especially chains, to shake the salt. That's because many of the ingredients are purchased in bulk from food vendors. The items are cheap and highly processed; thus, they are preserved with salt. Until suppliers begin reducing sodium in their items, restaurants won't be able to achieve much success when attempting to lower the sodium content in meals, unless, of course, they prepare the meals from scratch.

According to CNBC news, the average sodium content of all items among the biggest chain in 2014 was 1,256 milligrams. This means if your recommended sodium intake is 1,500 milligrams per day, you'd be close to your recommended level for the day after eating one meal.[9]

In 2016, *Forbes* released an article, "The Nine Worst Restaurant Meals in America for 2016," exposing popular restaurants and the eye-opening sodium levels in their popular dishes. For example, the giant chipotle cheese steak from Jersey Mike's Subs has 4,330 milligrams of sodium. Yuck. The fried chicken and waffles benedict from The Cheesecake Factory contains 3,390 milligrams of sodium. Hello, kidney overdrive. When dining out, you can always look up the sodium content and other nutritional values of meals with free apps such as Restaurant Nutrition.

The chances of getting a low-sodium meal at a restaurant are increased if you go to a small, family-owned restaurant that takes pride in their ingredients. If they promote that all the dishes and ingredients are made from scratch or in house, then there is a good chance their meals don't have sky-high sodium content. Moreover, you can most likely ask for no added salt without an issue. That brings us to the number one tip when dining out: Stay away from chains and fast-food restaurants.

Controlling your sodium should not spoil the pleasure and relaxation of dining out. Rather, think of it as adopting new habits into your lifestyle to preserve your health (and not reverse all of your hard work of eating healthy during the week). If you are familiar with low-sodium foods, you should have no trouble looking for them on the menu. Also, don't be afraid to get specific with your server about how you want your food prepared. Say things such as, "Can I please have that without added salt?" Servers, chefs, and restaurants are getting very good at complying with special dietary requests. Also, you can always add fresh lemon juice or an olive oil and garlic mixture to fish and veggies instead of salt. You

---

9   Katie Little, "Can't Shake the Salt? Worst Restaurant Offenders," CNBC. June 11, 2015, https://www.cnbc.com/2015/06/11/just-how-much-sodium-do-restaurant-meals-have.html.

can even ask for some ground garlic or another beloved spice/herb to add to your food.

Here are additional tips for eating out while on the DASH diet:

1. Skip the bread. You've heard it a million times, but there is a reason for this! It's a filler food that turns into pure sugar in your body. Don't spoil your appetite or fill up on bread by indulging too much before the meal. I know, I know. It's habit. You might even go to a certain restaurant specifically for their bread. But eating balanced meals beforehand should prevent the desire to munch on bread, since your blood sugar levels will be more stable. Thus, you won't feel that you *need* the bread. That brings me to an important rule: Never go to a restaurant starving. Also, as soon as you sit down, make it easier on yourself and ask the server not to bring bread, but rather a small salad.

2. Keep it simple and balanced. Don't order fried food or pasta. You will feel much better if you do this. Besides, eating delicious, healthy, balanced meals at a restaurant is possible *and* tastes good. Choose a meat or other source of protein (about 4 to 5 ounces), a starch such as brown rice (or white rice if you're on potassium restriction), and unlimited non-starchy veggies! Top it all off with a healthy fat, such as a side of avocado or olive oil. Many restaurant dishes follow this trend (protein, starch, and veggie); however, the proteins and starches are usually oversized and the veggie is undersized. Customize your meal! Tell the server the portion sizes you want.

   Fish tends to taste great at restaurants, so if you don't eat it regularly, this is a perfect opportunity to get in your omega-3s! Here's some healthy, balanced lunch or dinner options:

   - Steak with a sweet potato and a side of broccoli with olive oil and garlic
   - A salad with chicken, avocado, and olive oil and balsamic dressing
   - Grilled salmon with broccoli and rice

- Garlic rosemary chicken with mashed potatoes and sautéed spinach

3. Avoid the inflammatory oils. Restaurants are notorious for using those inflammatory oils that wreak havoc internally (a list of oils to avoid are discussed on page 67). Why? Because they're cheap. And as you know, oftentimes restaurants seek profit, not consumer health. Keep it safe by sticking with olive oil and vinegar on salads. Choose foods that are steamed, grilled, or prepared using other cooking methods that don't involve heavy oil use.

4. Be innovative. Don't be afraid to ask for substitutions. For example, skip the toast and ask for an extra egg, veggies, or a side of fruit. If a certain sandwich sounds delicious, ask for it served over fresh greens instead of bread, or do an open sandwich (ask them to take the top slice of bread off). You can get creative by asking to add avocado to your salad. You can always bring your own avocado slices or quality dressing. Tip: Travel-size shampoo and conditioner containers are great for carrying olive oil.

5. Ask for water. Ordering water saves you from drinking tablespoon upon tablespoon of unnecessary sugar. If you insist on ordering a beverage, seltzer is a refreshing option free of sugar and artificial sweetener. Ask for added oranges, lemons, and limes to give it natural flavor. Unsweetened tea and coffee are good options, too.

6. Plan ahead. Planning ahead not only reduces the stress and panic some feel when ordering at a restaurant, but it's very wise to do for those who are new to a healthy-eating lifestyle. Do your research prior to arriving at the restaurant by checking out their menu online. Decide what you'll order beforehand to avoid the temptation of choosing pasta or fried dishes.

7. Split food and take home leftovers. Go halves with your partner or friend if you must get an appetizer or dessert, especially if you rarely go out to eat. All foods can fit into a healthy diet when

eaten in moderation! If you're going to get an appetizer, don't go for a dessert. Try to choose one or the other, because consuming an appetizer, entrée, and dessert is one way to take in an entire day's worth of calories (and sodium!).

When your meal comes, ask the server to give you a container. That way you can immediately pack up half to go home and avoid the temptation of eating more when you're probably already full. Only do this if the portion is large; otherwise, you may not feel full and be more tempted to order dessert.

Those are just a few ways to enjoy eating away from home without having to sacrifice your healthy lifestyle. See? Eating out is totally doable and simple.

# Supermarket Tips

Your trips to the supermarket shouldn't be another daunting task on your already-long to-do list. With our tips, your supermarket trips will be faster and more budget friendly, and you'll be bringing home the proper DASH foods. Heck, you may even begin to love your supermarket trips, which tends to happen to our clients with their newfound love of healthy eating. Once you start understanding how to read labels, what food items you're looking for, and why healthy eating is so important, you'll take food shopping more seriously and you'll be interested in finding new healthy foods to trial and cook with.

Refer to this guide when developing your food shopping list (also see page 184 for a Food Shopping List you can copy and use). Let's face it: It is much easier to eat healthy at home when your fridge and pantries are stocked with the right foods. If you can avoid purchasing the not-so-healthy foods while grocery shopping, due to increased awareness and your food shopping list, you'll be more inclined to comply with the DASH diet at home. Saying no to that bag of chips or box of cookies in the grocery store goes a long way and it is a lot easier than saying no when it's in your pantry. Fight the temptation in the grocery aisle, keep on walking, and focus on your list and what foods you need to purchase to properly fuel your body and keep diseases at bay.

When food shopping, keep in mind it's best to purchase "clean foods," or foods that are whole, unprocessed, and as close as nature intended the food to be. Foods and beverages with artificial colors or flavors, added sugar, preservatives, additives, and chemical-laden ingredients are not included (usually packaged foods with long ingredient lists). With up to 42,000 food items available at a typical supermarket, choosing foods that will best support your health may seem tricky. It's important not to fall for advertisements, health claims, and foods that "look" healthy. For example, the front package of a food or beverage product may say "no artificial colors!"; however, the product includes artificial flavors. Do not get fooled! Food companies are great at tricking people into thinking it's a healthy product with misleading claims. This is why the best thing to do to find out what's in a food product is to read the ingredient list.

Online shopping and food delivery is becoming wildly popular. For fresh food, such as produce, it's best to purchase locally from a farmers market or your local grocery store to limit your food's additional travel time. However, getting staple foods delivered, such as dried spices and herbs, oils, beans, pastas, rice, and more pantry items is convenient, decreases your grocery store bulk, and is usually cheaper online.

Thrive Market is an excellent online healthy food shop that delivers quality goods at 25%–50% off retail prices. Although there is a yearly membership fee, most members make the money back in their first few orders. Also, they usually ship free for orders over $49.00. Moreover, for each product, the brand is explained and the ingredients list and Nutrition Facts label is clearly listed. This makes reading food labels a heck of a lot easier. Nobody is bumping into you with their cart or giving you the stink eye. You can take your sweet time reading all about the ingredients and nutrition from the comfort of your own home. Amazon is another excellent place to buy staple foods online.

As you've learned, most whole foods are located around the perimeter of the grocery store. Start your shopping trip by walking the perimeter, picking up the bulk of the foods you need. Keep your list on hand and refer to it as needed. Try not to deviate from the items on your list. Many of the products in the middle aisles of the grocery store are processed, with extra salt, bad fats, sugar, preservatives, and artificial ingredients. You should only be going into the middle aisles for staple foods, such as oils, rice, healthy pastas, and other items of that nature.

While deli meats are convenient for lunch, many are highly processed and contain significant amounts of sodium, nitrates, and even sugar. The same is true for hot dog and sausages. Purchase Applegate brand deli meats, bacon, and sausages, as these meats contain no antibiotics or hormones, have simple ingredients, and contain nothing artificial. Be aware of serving sizes, as these food products still contain high sodium compared to other foods.

When purchasing breads, cereals, and grains, find products that are minimally processed, contain no artificial colors (such as caramel coloring), contain low or no added sugar, and provides at least 3 grams of fiber per serving. A good pasta choice is Banza chickpea pasta, as it has high protein and fiber content. Many other lentil- or bean-based pastas are high in fiber and protein. We find that most of our patients like the taste of the bean- or chickpea- based pastas compared to wheat pastas.

Like most foods in the middle aisles of the supermarket, most frozen food products are highly processed, such as microwavable dinners. Do not purchase frozen veggies in sauces because they have tons of sodium and a much longer ingredients list. However, plain frozen fruits and vegetables are fine, as they only have one ingredient!

Plain frozen fruits and veggies are usually picked at peak season and have better nutrient retention. Fresh produce usually has greater nutrient loss due to sensitivities to light and oxygen. Stock up on plain frozen fruits and veggies to have on hand for when you run out of fresh produce, to add to smoothies, or for a quick microwavable veggie. Microwavable veggies are great for bulking up meals. For example, if you come home to a big bowl of pasta made by your significant other, friend, or family member, then you can choose to eat half of that but quickly microwave broccoli to pair it with. This will keep the sodium content of your meal down while adding tons of nutrients. Plus, you'll probably sleep better without having had a plain bowl of pasta for dinner.

Purchasing the right seasonings and condiments makes your food taste good and can even add an antioxidant boost (thanks to dried herbs and spices). Some condiments can have a lot of chemicals in them, so be sure to purchase those with small ingredients lists, such as vinegars, honey, maple syrup, mustard, and chicken stock. What's more, if you make your own dressings and sauces, you can keep them stored in jars in the fridge. This is something that shouldn't take too long, can last at least a few weeks, and is much better for your health.

# Stocking the Pantry

It's a good idea to have a week or two's worth of ingredients handy. This will help prevent you from reaching for quick—and often unhealthy—snacks or fast foods. While it's impossible to be prepared for everything, try to have some of these essentials stocked in your pantry, kitchen, and freezer. For example, if you have low-sodium broth and frozen veggies, you could throw together a quick soup. Or, if you have low-sodium canned beans and quinoa, you can make a meal in under 15 minutes. Skim through the recommended foods and recipes sections and take note of any favorites you'd like to include. Here are some recommended brands:

Applegate (cheese, turkey bacon, deli meals)

Banza (chickpea pasta)

Bragg's (apple cider vinegar, liquid aminos)

Bob's Red Mill (flour, oats)

Food For Life/Ezekiel (wraps, English muffins, bread)

Frontier (herbs and spices)

Jovial (brown rice pasta, flours)

Sir Kensington's (ketchup, mayonnaise)

Vital Farms (grass-fed butter, pasture-raised eggs)

We've discussed that many salt substitutes have potassium chloride, which can also be an unhealthy and dangerous alternative. Try some of these spices, herbs, oils, and acids for added flavor instead:

Basil

Cardamom

Cayenne pepper

Chili powder

Chilis and peppers (as mild or hot as you like)

Chives

Cilantro

Cinnamon, ground and sticks

Citrus juice: lemon, lime, orange

Citrus zest: lemon, lime, orange

Cloves

Coriander, ground

Cumin, ground

Curry powder

Dill

Garlic, raw or roasted

Ginger

Herbs de Provence

Infused oils (basil-infused olive oil, truffle oil, and chili oil are a few examples)

Mint

Oregano

Onions, raw or caramelized (these can add an umami, or fat, flavor)

Parsley

Rosemary

Thyme

Vinegar: apple cider, balsamic, rice, red wine, white wine, champagne

## Chapter 6
# RECIPES

You've done it. You've read all about the science behind the DASH diet and kidney health. You know what to eat, what to avoid, how the DASH diet can help your kidney health, and why. But you may be wondering how to make meals out of your newfound nutrition plan. In this section, we've created some recipes that are DASH- and kidney-health friendly, as well as some Sample Meal Plans (page 180) as examples for ways you can put them together in a day. If a recipe is high in a certain nutrient, such as potassium, we let you know. That way, it is up to you to swap it out with a lower potassium food or cut the ingredient out completely.

You now have all the tools you need to be successful on the DASH diet. Congratulations! Make a special homemade meal chosen from the following recipes to celebrate your new lifestyle—and your new commitment to a lifetime of good health and longevity.

Recipe Tips:

• All the recipes are low sodium.

• Be mindful of nuts: They're high in potassium and phosphorous.

• Use white rice and pastas when you need to limit phosphorous.

• Use cheese sparingly when reducing sodium and phosphorous.

• Adjust the amount of meat for a lower or higher protein content.

• Cooking your own beans will greatly reduce the sodium content of recipes compared to buying canned beans.

# BREAKFAST

## French Toast

3 eggs

½ cup unsweetened hemp, coconut, or almond milk

½ teaspoon vanilla extract

½ teaspoon ground cinnamon

¼ teaspoon ground nutmeg

1 tablespoon maple syrup, plus more to top (optional)

2 tablespoons grass-fed butter

8 slices Ezekiel cinnamon raisin bread

fresh fruit, to top (optional)

chopped walnuts, to top (optional)

1. In a shallow bowl, mix the eggs, milk, vanilla, cinnamon, nutmeg, and maple syrup.

2. Add the butter to a pan or griddle over medium heat.

3. Dip a slice of bread in the batter, coating each side but working quickly so that the bread doesn't get soggy.

4. Place the battered bread on the pan and cook 2 to 3 minutes until golden brown. Flip and repeat on the other side.

5. Repeat for each slice, or work in batches.

6. Top with a dash of maple syrup, fresh fruit, and chopped walnuts, if desired, or eat it plain.

*Serves:* 4

*Prep time:* 10 minutes

*Cooking time:* 20 minutes

# Banana Oat Shake

If you are limiting your potassium, use fresh or frozen berries or apples in place of a banana.

½ cup cooked oatmeal, chilled

½ frozen banana, cut into chunks

⅔ cup milk of choice

1 tablespoon maple syrup

½ teaspoon vanilla extract

1 tablespoon nut butter

handful ice

Place ingredients in blender. Blend until smooth.

*Serves:* 1

*Prep time:* 5 minutes

*Cooking time:* 0 minutes

# English Muffin Pizza

1 Ezekiel English muffin, cut in half

¼ cup pizza sauce

2 tablespoons shredded mozzarella cheese

sautéed broccoli, onions, or other veggies, to top (optional)

1.  Toast English muffins.

2.  Spread pizza sauce evenly on muffin halves.

3.  Sprinkle cheese and add optional toppings.

4.  Place the muffin halves on tray and put in the oven to broil for approximately 5 minutes.

5.  Add additional toppings, such as broccoli, if desired.

*Serves:* 1

*Prep time:* 5 minutes

*Cooking time:* 5 minutes

# Minimal Ingredient Banana Pancakes

Not an ideal choice when restricting potassium.

1 ripe medium banana, mashed

2 eggs

2½ teaspoons coconut flour

pinch baking powder

pinch ground cinnamon

¼ teaspoon coconut oil, for greasing

chia seeds, nut butter, or walnuts, to top

1. In a medium bowl, mash the banana down with a fork. Then add the eggs, coconut flour, baking powder, and cinnamon, and mix to combine.

2. Heat a skillet over medium heat. Grease it with coconut oil.

3. Spoon ⅛ cup of the batter onto the skillet for each pancake.

4. Cook until the surface of the pancakes bubble and sides firm up, about 2 minutes.

5. Carefully flip the pancakes with a spatula. Cook the underside for another 1 to 2 minutes.

6. Transfer the pancakes to a platter and serve with chia seeds, nut butter, or walnuts.

*Serves:* 2

*Prep time:* 5 minutes

*Cooking time:* 10 minutes

# Veggie Omelet

2 tablespoons grass-fed butter

½ cup chopped red bell pepper

½ cup chopped sweet yellow onion

½ cup chopped mushrooms

8 eggs

2 sliced avocados, to serve

1. Add the butter to a large pan. Heat to medium.

2. Add the vegetables to the pan. Cook for 4 to 5 minutes, stirring occasionally, until they are just tender. Remove and set aside.

3. In a medium bowl, whisk the eggs until well beaten.

4. To make the first of four omelets, add a quarter of the egg mixture to the pan that the vegetables were in. Let it cook for 2 minutes or until the eggs begin to set. Gently lift the edges of the omelet with a small spatula and tilt the pan slightly to let the uncooked part of the eggs flow toward the edges. Cook 2 more minutes.

5. Add ¼ of the veggie mixture to one half of the partially cooked egg mixture.

6. Using the spatula, fold the other side of the egg on top, making a pocket. Let it set for 1 minute. Remove from heat.

7. Repeat with remaining three omelets.

8. Plate each omelet with half an avocado, sliced.

*Serves:* 4

*Prep time:* 10 minutes

*Cooking time:* 10 minutes

# Lemon Blueberry Muffins

The local honey in this recipe is excellent for those with allergies.

1 tablespoon grass-fed butter

2¼ cups coconut flour

2 teaspoons baking soda

1 teaspoon baking powder

pinch Himalayan sea salt

1 lemon, juice and zest

⅔ cup unsweetened coconut milk

1 teaspoon vanilla extract

⅔ cup local honey

½ cup grapeseed oil

1 cup fresh blueberries, divided

1. Grease a 12-cup muffin tin with the butter.

2. Preheat the oven to 350°F.

3. In a large bowl, whisk together the flour, baking soda, baking powder, and salt, and set aside.

4. In a medium bowl, whisk together the lemon zest and juice, milk, vanilla, and honey. Once combined, slowly whisk in the oil.

5. Add the wet mixture to the dry, and mix until combined. Don't overmix.

6. Gently fold in ⅔ cup of blueberries.

7. Scoop the batter into the muffin pan. Top the muffins with the remaining ⅓ of cup blueberries.

8. Bake for 18 to 20 minutes or until a toothpick inserted into the center of a muffin comes out clean.

*Serves:* 12

*Prep time:* 15 minutes

*Cooking time:* 20 minutes

# Berry Overnight Oats

Substitute steel cut oats with cream of wheat if you have a phosphorous restriction.

1 cup unsweetened coconut milk or water

1 cup frozen strawberries

1½ cups steel cut oats

¼ cup fresh strawberries

¼ cup fresh blueberries

1.  In a blender, blend the water or milk and frozen strawberries.

2.  Divide the oats evenly into two sealable containers or jars.

3.  Pour half the strawberry/milk mixture into each jar. Stir the contents of each jar to mix ingredients.

4.  Cover and refrigerate overnight (or at least 6 hours).

5.  When you're ready to enjoy, top with fresh strawberries and blueberries. Serve cold.

*Serves:* 2
*Prep time:* 5 minutes
*Cooking time:* 0 minutes

# Nutty Overnight Oats

Not a good choice when restricting phosphorous.

½ cup unsweetened coconut milk or water

¾ tablespoon chia seeds

2 tablespoons salt-free peanut butter or almond butter

½ tablespoon maple syrup

½ cup quick cooking oats

chopped fruit, to garnish (optional)

1. To a mason jar or small bowl, add the milk or water, chia seeds, nut butter, and maple syrup. Stir with a spoon to combine. Don't completely mix the peanut butter with the milk so as to leave delicious swirls of peanut butter.

2. Add the oats and stir a few more times. Press down with a spoon to ensure all oats have been immersed in milk.

3. Cover securely with a lid or plastic wrap.

4. Cover and refrigerate overnight (or at least 6 hours).

5. Before serving, garnish with chopped fruit, if desired. Serve cold.

*Serves:* 1
*Prep time:* 5 minutes
*Cooking time:* 0 minutes

# Homemade Blueberry Muesli

2 cups steel cut oats

1 cup rolled spelt

½ cup dried blueberries

½ cup chopped almonds

½ cup chopped pecans

¼ cup ground flaxseed

2 tablespoons local honey

½ teaspoon ground cinnamon

1. Preheat the oven to 350°F.

2. In a large bowl, combine the oats, spelt, blueberries, almonds, pecans, and flaxseed. Mix well.

3. Pour in the honey and toss to coat evenly. Sprinkle with cinnamon and toss well.

4. Pour the mixture evenly onto a baking sheet and bake for 15 minutes, stirring once halfway.

5. Remove from the heat and let cool.

*Serves:* 14 to 16

*Prep time:* 5 minutes

*Cooking time:* 15 minutes

# Greek Yogurt Parfait

Use coconut or almond milk yogurt when restricting potassium.

1 cup plain Greek yogurt, divided

1 cup homemade or store-bought muesli, divided

½ cup fresh blueberries, divided

½ tablespoon walnuts, divided

1 tablespoon chia seeds, divided

1. Layer ¼ cup of the yogurt on the bottom of a mason jar, small bowl, or cup.

2. Top with ¼ cup of the muesli, then ⅛ cup of blueberries, ⅛ tablespoon walnuts, and ¼ tablespoon chia seeds.

3. Repeat layering yogurt, muesli, fruit, walnuts, and chia seeds until the ingredients run out.

*Serves:* 1

*Prep time:* 5 minutes

*Cooking time:* 0 minutes

# LUNCH/DINNER

## Beef Barley Soup

2 pounds beef stew meat, cut into 1-inch cubes

½ teaspoon black pepper

4 tablespoons grapeseed oil

1 cup chopped onion

1 cup sliced carrots

1 cup sliced mushrooms

½ teaspoon minced garlic

¼ teaspoon dried thyme

1 (14.5-ounce) can low-sodium chicken or bone broth

3 cups water

16 ounces frozen or fresh mixed veggies

2 soaked potatoes, diced

½ cup barley

1. Season beef with pepper.

2. Add the oil to a stew pot. Warm it over medium heat.

3. Add the onion, carrots, and mushrooms. Sauté for 5 minutes and stir often.

4. Add garlic and thyme. Sauté for 3 minutes.

5. Add chicken broth and water. Add mixed vegetables, potatoes, and barley. Stir and bring to a boil. Cover and reduce heat.

6. Simmer for 1 to 1½ hours.

*Serves:* 10
*Prep time:* 15 minutes
*Cooking time:* 1 to 2 hours

# Lemony Vegetable and Rice Salad

Limit tomatoes with potassium restriction.

1¼ cups uncooked white or brown rice

½ pound fresh asparagus, trimmed and chopped

1 medium zucchini, sliced into discs

1 serving Lemon Vinaigrette (page 158)

1 portobello mushroom, stem removed, sliced

1 medium yellow, orange, or red bell pepper, seeded and sliced

¼ medium red onion, sliced into strips

1 cup halved grape or cherry tomatoes

1 tablespoon chopped fresh parsley

1 tablespoon chopped fresh basil

¼ teaspoon pepper

1 tablespoon lemon juice

1. Cook rice according to package instructions. Set aside.

2. Place chopped asparagus and zucchini in a large bowl. Add the Lemon Vinaigrette dressing to the vegetables and toss to coat evenly.

3. Drain the extra dressing into a small cup or bowl. Use it to coat the mushroom, pepper, and onion, and then sauté them in a large pan over medium heat for 5 to 7 minutes or until they're tender, stirring occasionally.

4. Add the asparagus and zucchini and cook for another 3 to 4 minutes or until they reach desired doneness, stirring occasionally. Remove from heat and transfer to a large bowl to let cool.

5. In a separate large bowl, combine the cooked rice, cooked vegetables, tomatoes, parsley, basil, and pepper.

6. Sprinkle with lemon juice and toss to combine. Serve at room temperature. Refrigerate for up to 3 days.

*Serves:* 8
*Prep time:* 20 minutes
*Cooking time:* 15 minutes

# Fiesta Lime Ground Turkey

For lower phosphorous, switch from corn tortillas to white flour tortillas.

1 pound ground turkey

4 tablespoons Mrs. Dash Fiesta Lime Seasoning Blend

¾ cup water

12 corn tortillas

sliced radishes, cilantro, and finely chopped onion, to top (optional)

1. Brown the ground meat in a large skillet over medium heat, about 15 minutes. Drain excess fat.

2. Stir in Mrs. Dash Fiesta Lime Seasoning Blend and water.

3. Bring to a boil. Reduce heat and simmer 5 minutes, stirring occasionally.

4. Spoon turkey into warm corn tortillas. Serve with desired toppings.

*Serves:* 12
*Prep time:* 5 minutes
*Cooking time:* 20 minutes

# Slow Cooker Chicken and White Bean Chili

1 pound boneless, skinless chicken breast, cut into bite-sized cubes

1 teaspoon black pepper

4 cups low-sodium chicken broth or bone broth

1 cup white beans, from can

6 pearl onions

¾ cup diced onion

¾ cup diced carrots

¾ cup diced celery

4 cloves garlic, minced

2 teaspoons garlic powder

2 teaspoons ground cumin

2 teaspoons chili powder

1 teaspoon dried oregano

¼ teaspoon cayenne pepper

1. Season chicken with black pepper and place in a slow cooker.

2. Rinse and drain beans to reduce sodium.

3. Add chicken broth or bone broth, beans, pearl onions, diced onion, carrots, celery, and garlic to slow cooker.

4. Season with garlic powder, cumin, chili powder, oregano, and cayenne pepper.

5. Cover with lid and cook on low setting for 8 hours.

*Serves:* 8
*Prep time:* 10 minutes
*Cooking time:* 8 hours

# Spicy Baked Fish

Optionally, serve with ½ cup of brown rice or cauliflower rice. For cauliflower rice, buy it frozen and sauté it in a pan with 1 to 2 tablespoons of grapeseed oil for 15 minutes. For brown rice, follow the cooking instructions on the box. For lower phosphorous, switch from cod to mahi mahi.

| | |
|---|---|
| 2 tablespoons coconut oil, divided | 1 teaspoon salt-free spicy seasoning |
| 1 pound cod fillet | |

1. Preheat the oven to 350°F.

2. Melt 1 tablespoon coconut oil and then add to casserole dish.

3. Wash and dry fish. Place in a dish and mix with 1 tablespoon oil and seasoning.

4. Bake uncovered for 15 minutes or until fish flakes with a fork.

5. Cut into 4 pieces to serve.

*Serves:* 4

*Prep time:* 5 minutes

*Cooking time:* 15 minutes

# Pear and Cranberry Salad with Honey-Ginger Dressing

2 cups watercress

4 cups baby green leaf lettuce

1 medium pear, roughly chopped

⅓ cup dried cranberries

2 tablespoons chopped pecans

2 tablespoons apple cider vinegar

1 tablespoon local honey

¼ cup extra virgin olive oil

2 teaspoons ginger paste or minced ginger

1 teaspoon Dijon mustard

1. In a large bowl, combine the watercress, lettuce, pear, cranberries, and pecan pieces.

2. In a jar, combine the vinegar, honey, olive oil, ginger, and mustard.

3. Cover the jar with a lid and shake until the dressing is well mixed.

4. Pour the dressing over the salad and toss.

*Serves:* 6
*Prep time:* 10 minutes
*Cooking time:* 0 minutes

# Spinach Salad

Use only arugula when restricting potassium. Green or red leaf lettuce are also lower potassium greens you may use.

3 cups baby spinach

3 cups arugula

½ cup chopped pecans

2½ cups sliced fresh strawberries

¼ cup goat cheese, crumbled

½ avocado, diced

2 tablespoons olive oil

½ lemon, juiced

1. In a large bowl, toss the spinach and arugula together to combine.

2. Toast the pecans in a small skillet over medium-low heat for 2 to 3 minutes, or until slightly browned. Be careful not to burn them. Remove from heat and set aside.

3. Top greens mixture with strawberries, toasted pecans, goat cheese, and avocado. Drizzle with olive oil and lemon juice, or Balsamic Dijon Dressing (page 158). Toss to combine.

*Serves:* 4
*Prep time:* 10 minutes
*Cooking time:* 3 minutes

# Pesto Potato Salad

Not a good choice for those restricting potassium.

*For the potato salad:*

1 pound (6 to 8) small red-skinned potatoes

2 teaspoons fresh lemon juice

2 cups fresh green beans, trimmed and halved

¼ cup chopped raw walnuts

*For the pesto:*

½ avocado, sliced

1 clove garlic, minced

1 cup fresh basil

3 cups baby arugula

2 tablespoons raw walnuts

½ lemon, juiced

1 tablespoon olive oil

black pepper, to taste

1. Bring a medium pot of water to a boil over high heat. Add the potatoes and lemon juice, then lower the heat to a simmer. Cook for 10 to 15 minutes, or until tender.

2. Transfer to a bowl to cool using a slotted spoon, leaving the water to simmer.

3. Add the green beans to the pot and cook for 5 minutes.

4. Transfer the green beans to a separate bowl.

5. Rinse both the potatoes and green beans in cold water and then drain.

6. Cut the potatoes to bite-size. Set aside.

7. For the pesto, combine the avocado, garlic, basil, arugula, 2 tablespoons walnuts, lemon juice, and olive oil in a food processor or high-speed blender and blend until smooth. Set aside.

8. To complete the salad, toss the potatoes and green beans with the ¼ cup chopped raw walnuts.

*Serves:* 4 to 6

*Prep time:* 10 minutes

*Cooking time:* 20 minutes

# Couscous and Veggies

1 tablespoon grapeseed oil

2 portobello mushrooms or ½ pound other mushrooms, chopped, stems removed

1 medium zucchini, chopped

1 medium red bell pepper, seeded and chopped

¼ cup white wine

2 tablespoons lemon juice

3 tablespoons Dijon mustard

2 tablespoons olive oil

2 cloves garlic, minced

¼ teaspoon black pepper

1 cup water

1 cup uncooked couscous

2 tablespoons chopped fresh basil

1. Preheat the oven to 350°F. Add grapeseed oil to a baking dish. Set aside.

2. In a large bowl, combine the vegetables.

3. In a small bowl, whisk together the wine, lemon juice, mustard, olive oil, garlic, and pepper.

4. Drizzle the dressing over the vegetables and toss to coat evenly. Pour them into the baking dish.

5. Bake for 20 to 25 minutes or until vegetables are tender. Remove from the oven and set aside to cool.

6. In a small pot, bring water to a boil. Stir in the couscous and remove immediately from heat. Cover it and let it stand for 5 to 10 minutes or until the water is absorbed. Fluff it lightly with a fork.

7. Transfer the couscous and vegetables to a large bowl and toss to combine. Sprinkle with fresh basil. Serve.

*Serves:* 4

*Prep time:* 20 minutes

*Cooking time:* 25 minutes

# Lemon Rosemary Chicken Skillet

1 pint grape or cherry tomatoes

1½ teaspoons black pepper, divided

1 tablespoon plus 1 teaspoon grapeseed oil

4 boneless, skinless chicken breasts

1½ teaspoons dried rosemary, divided

½ cup white wine

2 cloves garlic, minced

1 lemon, juiced

1. Preheat the oven to 400°F.

2. In a medium bowl, toss the tomatoes with half of the pepper and one teaspoon of grapeseed oil.

3. Place the tomatoes in a cast-iron skillet (or, if you don't have one, a baking dish) and roast for 15 minutes.

4. While the tomatoes are roasting, pat the chicken dry with paper towels. Season with ½ teaspoon rosemary and half of remaining pepper.

5. Remove the tomatoes from the oven, but keep the oven on. Remove the tomatoes from the skillet and set aside, and place the skillet on a burner set to medium-high. If you don't have a cast-iron skillet, switch to a large skillet.

6. Coat the skillet with the remaining grapeseed oil. Once it's hot, place the chicken into the skillet. Let it sear, and turn after 2 minutes. Sear for 1 minute. Remove the chicken from the pan and set aside.

7. With the pan still on medium high heat, pour the white wine in. It will hiss and bubble a bit. Let it settle. While stirring, add the garlic, remaining rosemary, and remaining pepper. Add the juice from the lemon. Stir occasionally, and let it cook for 2 to 3 minutes.

8. If you're using a cast-iron skillet, return the chicken right to the skillet. If you're using a regular skillet and baking dish, add the chicken to the baking dish and then pour the sauce mixture over the chicken and tomatoes. Place the skillet or dish in the oven.

9.  Bake for 30 minutes or until the chicken is cooked through and opaque.

10. Remove from the oven. Serve the chicken topped with the tomatoes.

*Serves:* 4
*Prep time:* 15 minutes
*Cooking time:* 60 minutes

# Grilled Chicken Paillard

4 boneless, skinless chicken breasts

2 tablespoons olive oil

½ teaspoon black pepper

¼ teaspoon garlic powder

½ tablespoon dried basil

1 lemon, cut into 4 wedges, to serve

½ teaspoon dried parsley, to serve

1. Preheat the grill to medium-high.

2. Place each chicken breast between 2 sheets of wax paper or plastic wrap. Using a meat mallet or a similar utensil, pound the chicken evenly until it is approximately ¼-inch thick.

3. Lightly brush both sides of each chicken breast with olive oil.

4. In a small bowl, combine the pepper, garlic powder, and basil, and sprinkle it evenly over both sides of the chicken breasts.

5. Grill the chicken about 8 minutes, turning once halfway through, until browned and cooked through.

6. Serve. Sprinkle with parsley and serve with lemon wedges.

*Serves*: 4

*Prep time*: 10 minutes

*Cooking time*: 15 minutes

# Spiced Chicken

2 teaspoons paprika

1 teaspoon ground cumin

1 teaspoon dried thyme

1 teaspoon garlic powder

¼ cup balsamic vinegar

1 tablespoon local honey

4 boneless, skinless chicken breasts

salt and pepper, to taste

1. Preheat the oven to 425°F.

2. In a small bowl, combine the paprika, cumin, thyme, and garlic. In another small bowl, whisk together the vinegar and honey.

3. Season the chicken with salt and pepper on both sides. Place the chicken in a baking dish, and pour the honey mixture over the chicken to coat. Then coat the chicken with the seasoning mixture on both sides.

4. Bake for 25 to 30 minutes, or until cooked through.

*Serves:* 4

*Prep time:* 10 minutes

*Cooking time:* 30 minutes

# Colorful Pizza

1 cup full-fat ricotta cheese

½ cup full-fat mozzarella cheese

¼ teaspoon dried basil

¼ teaspoon red pepper flakes

1 tablespoon grapeseed oil

½ medium sweet yellow onion, chopped

½ medium orange or yellow bell pepper, seeded and sliced into strips

1 portobello mushroom, stem removed, sliced

½ cup all-purpose flour

1 pound pizza dough, left out at room temperature for 1 hour

2 teaspoons olive oil

½ pint halved grape or cherry tomatoes

½ cup fresh spinach

⅓ cup fresh basil, to top

1. Place the oven rack at the middle and preheat the oven to 525°F.

2. In a small bowl, combine the ricotta, mozzarella, dried basil, and red pepper flakes, and set aside.

3. Heat the grapeseed oil in a medium skillet over medium-high heat. Add the onion, bell pepper, and mushroom. Cook for 5 to 7 minutes, stirring occasionally, until the vegetables start to become tender. Remove from heat and set aside.

4. Lightly flour a clean countertop or table, a rolling pin, and your hands. Roll out the pizza dough to fit your baking sheet.

5. Carefully transfer the dough to the baking sheet, then use your fingers to gently press the dough into the corners of the pan. Lightly coat the dough with olive oil.

6. Spread the cheese mixture over the dough, leaving about a ½-inch border around the edges. Spread the vegetables over the top, leaving the spinach for last.

7. Bake until the edges are golden brown, 16 to 20 minutes. Remove from the heat and immediately sprinkle with fresh basil.

8. Let cool for 1 to 2 minutes before cutting into slices and serving.

*Serves:* 4
*Prep time:* 20 minutes
*Cooking time:* 30 minutes

# Pasta Primavera

Banza chickpea pasta, brown rice pasta, or black bean pasta are preferred for this recipe, but for lower phosphorous content, use white pasta. For lower potassium, remove the tomatoes.

2 cups chopped broccoli

1 cup halved cherry or grape tomatoes

1 cup chopped portobello mushrooms

1 orange or yellow bell pepper, cored and chopped

5 tablespoons olive oil, divided

1 teaspoon dried basil

salt and pepper, to taste

16 ounces pasta

cooking spray

3 cloves garlic, minced

¼ cup balsamic vinegar

handful fresh basil leaves, to serve

¾ cup nutritional yeast, or fresh, quality mozzarella cheese or vegan Parmesan, to serve

1. Preheat the oven to 450°F. In a large bowl, toss the broccoli, tomatoes, mushrooms, and bell pepper with 3 tablespoons of olive oil and season with dried basil, salt, and pepper. Bake for 15 to 20 minutes.

2. Cook the pasta according to package instructions until it's al dente, about 8 minutes. Drain the pasta and reserve 1 cup of pasta water.

3. Coat a large pan with cooking spray. Cook the garlic over medium-high heat until browned. Add the drained pasta. Add a little bit of pasta water. Stir gently to combine. Add the roasted vegetables and stir.

4. Cook for 3 minutes, stirring occasionally, over medium heat, adding pasta water as needed.

5. Turn the heat to medium-high, cook for 1 more minute, and then pour the balsamic vinegar over the mixture. Give it one final stir and remove from heat.

6. Serve with fresh basil and vegan Parmesan, nutritional yeast, or mozzarella cheese.

*Serves:* 4
*Prep time:* 15 minutes
*Cooking time:* 30 minutes

# Chicken and Asparagus Skillet

4 boneless, skinless chicken breasts

1 teaspoon dried oregano, divided

1 teaspoon black pepper, divided

1 tablespoon grapeseed oil

1 lemon, sliced into rounds

2 cloves garlic, minced

1 bunch asparagus, ends trimmed and chopped into bite-sized pieces

1 teaspoon dried parsley, to serve

1. Preheat the oven to 400°F.

2. Pat the chicken dry with paper towels and season with half of the oregano and pepper.

3. Coat a cast-iron skillet, or if you don't have one, a regular skillet, with the grapeseed oil, and heat it over medium high.

4. When the pan is hot, add the chicken. Sear for 2 minutes and then flip, searing the other side for 1 minute.

5. Remove from heat and add the lemon slices, garlic, and asparagus, and season with the remaining oregano and pepper. If you're not using a cast-iron skillet, switch ingredients into a baking dish.

6. Cook in the oven for 30 minutes, or until chicken is cooked through and opaque.

7. Remove from the oven. Sprinkle with parsley and serve.

*Serves:* 4

*Prep time:* 5 minutes

*Cooking time:* 45 minutes

# Walnut-Crusted Chicken

Not a good choice for those limiting phosphorous.

4 boneless, skinless chicken breasts

⅓ cup olive oil

¼ cup plus 3 tablespoons whole grain Dijon mustard, divided

¼ cup white wine

4 cloves garlic, minced

1 teaspoon dried thyme

2 cups raw walnuts, chopped

1 cup whole wheat or coconut flour

salt and pepper, to taste

2 tablespoons grapeseed oil

⅓ cup local honey

2 tablespoons dried parsley, to serve

1. Combine the chicken, olive oil, ¼ cup mustard, white wine, garlic, and thyme in an airtight container or sealed bag. Refrigerate for 4 hours or overnight.

2. When you're ready to cook, preheat the oven to 425°F.

3. Combine the walnuts, flour, salt, and pepper together in a shallow baking dish. Dip the chicken into the walnut mixture and coat it evenly. Set aside.

4. Heat 2 tablespoons of grapeseed oil in a large oven-safe skillet over medium-high heat. Add the chicken and cook for 2 minutes on each side.

5. Transfer the skillet to the oven and bake for 15 to 20 minutes, or until the chicken is cooked through.

6. Remove from the oven and let cool.

7. In a small bowl, whisk together the honey and 3 tablespoons remaining mustard. Drizzle over the chicken, sprinkle with parsley, and serve.

*Serves*: 4

*Prep time*: 4½ hours

*Cooking time*: 25 minutes

# Dijon Chicken

3 cloves garlic, minced

½ cup whole grain Dijon mustard

½ teaspoon paprika

2 tablespoons chopped fresh tarragon

4 boneless, skinless chicken breasts

½ lemon, juiced

1. Preheat the oven to 425°F.

2. In a small bowl, whisk together the garlic, mustard, paprika, and tarragon. Set aside.

3. Coat the chicken with the mustard mixture. Bake for 25 to 30 minutes or until cooked through. Sprinkle with lemon juice before serving.

*Serves:* 4

*Prep time:* 10 minutes

*Cooking time:* 30 minutes

# Vegetable Green Curry

Remove spinach if you are restricting potassium.

1 cup uncooked white rice

water, as needed

1 tablespoon grapeseed oil

1 small yellow onion, diced

1 tablespoon minced fresh ginger

4 cloves garlic, minced

10 stalks green asparagus, chopped into 2-inch segments, ends removed

3 carrots, peeled and chopped

2 tablespoons Thai green curry paste

1 (14-ounce) can coconut milk

1 teaspoon honey

2 cups spinach

fresh cilantro

red pepper, to taste

1. Cook the rice as directed, but with at least a cup more water than needed. Once cooked, remove from heat and drain most of the water, retaining about a cup. Return the rice to the pot. Cover and let it rest.

2. Heat the grapeseed oil in a large, deep skillet over medium heat. Sauté the onion, ginger, and garlic for 2 to 3 minutes. Add the asparagus and carrots and cook for 3 minutes, stirring often. Add the curry paste and cook, stirring often, for 2 more minutes.

3. Add the coconut milk into the pan, along with the honey and ½ cup of the water from the rice. Bring the pan to a simmer. Cook until the carrots are tender, about 10 more minutes.

4. Add the spinach into the mixture and cook for about 30 more seconds. Remove the curry from heat and season lightly with fresh cilantro and crushed red pepper flakes. Serve over rice.

*Serves:* 4

*Prep time:* 5 minutes

*Cooking time:* 30 minutes

# Grilled Salmon

4 salmon fillets

1 teaspoon ground cumin

1 teaspoon paprika

1 teaspoon onion powder

1 teaspoon chili powder, or to taste

1 teaspoon garlic powder

salt and pepper, to taste

1. Season salmon lightly with salt and pepper.

2. In a small bowl, mix the cumin, paprika, onion powder, chili powder, and garlic powder.

3. If grilling, preheat the grill to medium-high, or if using an oven, preheat to 375°F.

4. Rub spice mixture onto the salmon, and then grill or bake for up to 10 minutes, or until cooked through to desired temperature.

*Serves:* 4

*Prep time:* 10 minutes

*Cooking time:* 10 minutes

# Rainbow Trout

2 tablespoons coconut oil

4 rainbow trout fillets

2 large tomatoes, peeled, seeded, and chopped

4 cloves garlic, sliced thinly

1 teaspoon grapeseed oil

1 tablespoon dried thyme

1 teaspoon dried rosemary

1 lemon, sliced into quarters, to top

handful chopped fresh parsley, to top

1. Preheat the oven to 450°F.

2. Grease a baking dish with coconut oil then place the trout, skin side down.

3. In a medium bowl, combine the tomatoes, garlic, and 1 teaspoon of grapeseed oil. Spoon the mixture over the middle of each piece of trout. Season with thyme and rosemary.

4. Bake for 10 to 15 minutes. Serve with lemon wedges and parsley.

*Serves:* 4

*Prep time:* 15 minutes

*Cooking time:* 15 minutes

# Chicken Salad

3¼ cups cooked, cubed skinless chicken

¼ cup chopped celery

¼ cup chopped onion

1 tablespoon lemon juice

½ teaspoon Mrs. Dash Garlic and Herb Seasoning Blend or Himalayan sea salt

3 tablespoons avocado mayonnaise

In a large bowl, combine all ingredients and mix well.

*Serves:* 5
*Prep time:* 10 minutes
*Cooking time:* 0 minutes


# Egg Salad

2 tablespoons avocado mayonnaise

1 teaspoon dry mustard

½ teaspoon black pepper

3 boiled eggs, chopped

1 tablespoon regular pickle relish

paprika

1. Mix together mayonnaise, mustard, pepper, eggs, and pickle relish.

2. Sprinkle with paprika.

*Serves:* 8
*Prep time:* 10 minutes
*Cooking time:* 0 minutes

# Herbed Chicken and Sweet Potatoes Skillet

Remove potatoes or replace with summer squash if you have potassium restriction.

¼ cup grapeseed oil

4 boneless, skinless chicken breasts

2 sweet potatoes, chopped

1 tablespoon dried thyme

1½ teaspoons dried tarragon

1½ teaspoons dried rosemary

2 lemons, 1 juiced and 1 sliced for serving

6 cloves garlic, minced

1. Preheat the oven to 400°F.

2. Add grapeseed oil to a large cast-iron skillet and heat over medium-high.

3. Add the chicken to the skillet. Add the sweet potatoes. Add thyme, tarragon, and rosemary and stir well to combine.

4. Cook for 5 minutes, stirring the sweet potatoes occasionally, then flip the chicken.

5. Pour the lemon juice and garlic over the chicken and potatoes and cook for 5 minutes more, stirring occasionally.

6. Slice the remaining lemon and place the slices on top of the chicken. Bake for 30 minutes, or until the chicken is cooked through.

*Serves:* 10
*Prep time:* 30 minutes
*Cooking time:* 40 minutes

# Super Veggie Turkey Meatloaf

1 medium onion, peeled and chopped

3 carrots, peeled and chopped

6 cloves garlic

¼ cup fresh thyme

1 cup shiitake mushrooms

2 tablespoons extra virgin olive oil

2 teaspoons Himalayan sea salt, divided

½ cup quick-cooking oats

½ cup unsweetened hemp milk

2 teaspoons Dijon mustard

½ cup plus two tablespoons low-sodium ketchup

1 egg

2 pounds ground turkey

1. Preheat the oven to 375°F.

2. Line a large baking sheet with parchment paper.

3. Combine the onion, carrots, garlic, and thyme in a food processor. Process until minced. Transfer to a bowl.

4. Add shiitake mushrooms to the bowl of the food processor. Process until just minced and then set aside.

5. Heat the oil in a large skillet over medium heat. Add the onion-carrot mixture and cook for about 6 minutes or until onion is just about to soften. Add the minced shiitake mushrooms to the skillet. Season with 1 teaspoon of salt and cook for 5 to 6 minutes, or until both the onion are mushrooms are soft. Set aside to cool.

6. In a large bowl, combine the oats, hemp milk, Dijon mustard, 2 tablespoons of ketchup, egg, and remaining teaspoon of salt. Use your clean hands to mix the ingredients together. Add the sautéed vegetables and ground turkey, and mix until everything is well blended.

7. Place the turkey meatloaf on the baking sheet and shape into a rounded rectangle. Brush the top with ½ cup ketchup.

8. Bake for 50 to 55 minutes.

9. Remove turkey meatloaf from the oven and let it rest 15 minutes before serving.

*Serves:* 6
*Prep time:* 20 minutes
*Cooking time:* 65 minutes

# Fish Tacos

For lower phosphorous, switch from corn tortillas to white flour tortillas.

1 pound cod fillets

2 limes, 1 juiced and 1 sliced into wedges

1 garlic clove, minced

½ teaspoon ground cumin

½ teaspoon chili powder

¼ teaspoon black pepper

1 tablespoon olive oil

½ cup avocado mayonnaise

¼ cup sour cream

2 tablespoons milk of choice

1 cup shredded cabbage

½ cup chopped red onion

½ bunch fresh chopped cilantro

12 (6-inch) corn tortillas

1. Place fish fillets in a dish. Squeeze lime juice from half a lime over the fish. Sprinkle fish with minced garlic, cumin, chili powder, black pepper, and olive oil. Turn fillets to coat with marinade and refrigerate for 15 to 30 minutes.

2. Make salsa blanca by combining avocado mayo, sour cream, milk, and juice of half a lime. Stir to combine and place in fridge to chill.

3. Broil fish on high until flesh turns white and fish flakes easily—about 10 minutes.

4. Remove fish from oven, cool slightly, and flake into large pieces.

5. Heat corn tortillas in a pan over low-medium heat until soft and warm. Wrap them in a dish towel to keep them warm.

6. Place a piece of fish on a tortilla. Top with salsa blanca, cabbage, red onion, cilantro, and lime wedges.

*Serves:* 6

*Prep time:* 40 minutes

*Cooking time:* 10 minutes

# Lemon Dill Salmon

1 teaspoon coconut oil

2 cloves garlic, minced

4 (½-pound) salmon fillets

½ teaspoon dried dill

2 lemons, 1 sliced into 8 slices, 1 cut into wedges

1. Preheat the oven to 400°F.

2. In a small skillet, heat coconut oil over medium heat.

3. Add minced garlic and cook until fragrant, 30 seconds to 1 minute. Be careful not to burn it, as it will cook quickly.

4. Place the salmon in a nonstick baking dish (or spray with nonstick spray), skin side down.

5. Lightly spread the tops of salmon fillets evenly with garlic and dill, and top with two lemon slices each.

6. Place in the oven and bake, uncovered, for 10 to 12 minutes. Salmon will be done when you can see beads of fat begin to cluster and become opaque, and it is opaque in the center.

7. Remove from the oven and serve with lemon wedges.

*Serves*: 4

*Prep time*: 10 minutes

*Cooking time*: 13 minutes

# SIDES AND SAUCES

## Greek Yogurt Salad Dressing

8 ounces plain Greek yogurt

¼ cup mayonnaise

2 tablespoons chopped fresh chives

2 tablespoons chopped fresh dill

2 tablespoons lemon juice

Mix all ingredients in a medium bowl and refrigerate until ready to serve.

*Serves:* 8

*Prep time:* 5 minutes

*Cooking time:* 0 minutes

## Grilled Portobello Mushrooms

½ cup chopped shallots

2 tablespoons balsamic vinegar

2 tablespoons sesame oil

2 teaspoons low-sodium soy sauce

3 large portobello mushrooms

1. Mix shallots, vinegar, oil, and soy sauce in a shallow baking dish.

2. Place mushrooms in dish and marinate overnight in fridge.

3. Grill mushrooms 5 minutes on each side or until darkened.

*Serves:* 6

*Prep time:* 3 minutes, plus overnight to marinate

*Cooking time:* 5 minutes

# Colorful Steamed Squash

2 zucchini, ends cut, halved lengthwise, and cut into bite-sized half moons

2 summer squash, ends cut, halved lengthwise, and cut into bite-sized half moons

2 cloves garlic, minced

1 tablespoon olive oil

1. Bring a large pot of water to a boil.

2. Place the zucchini, squash, and garlic into a double boiler basket, then place the basket into the pot of boiling water. Cover and let steam for about 15 minutes, or until the vegetables are tender.

3. Remove from heat and place in a large bowl.

4. Drizzle evenly with the olive oil and toss to combine.

*Serves:* 4

*Prep time:* 5 minutes

*Cooking time:* 15 minutes

# Roasted Cauliflower

3 cloves garlic, minced

2 tablespoons olive oil

1 head cauliflower, chopped into bite-sized florets

1 tablespoon dried rosemary

½ tablespoon red pepper flakes

1 tablespoon dried parsley, to serve

2 tablespoons lemon juice, to serve

1. Preheat the oven to 450°F.

2. In a large bowl, combine the garlic, olive oil, and cauliflower.

3. Sprinkle with rosemary and red pepper flakes. Toss well to combine.

4. Pour mixture into a nonstick baking dish (or spray dish with nonstick spray).

5. Bake for 15 minutes and stir. Bake for another 15 minutes. Remove from heat.

6. Top with parsley and sprinkle with lemon juice to serve.

*Serves:* 6

*Prep time:* 15 minutes

*Cooking time:* 30 minutes

# Zucchini Bread

With potassium restriction, used dried cranberries instead of raisins.

| | |
|---|---|
| ⅓ cup maple syrup | 3 teaspoons ground cinnamon |
| 3 eggs, beaten | 2½ cups coconut flour |
| 3 teaspoons vanilla extract | ½ teaspoon baking powder |
| 1 teaspoon Himalayan sea salt | 2 cups grated zucchini |
| 1 teaspoon baking soda | ½ teaspoon cloves |
| ½ teaspoon ground nutmeg | ½ cup raisins (optional) |

1. Preheat the oven to 350°F.

2. Grease 2 loaf pans.

3. Mix all ingredients together in the order provided.

4. Pour into the pans.

5. Bake for 45 to 60 minutes until a toothpick inserted in the center comes out clean.

*Serves:* 14
*Prep time:* 15 minutes
*Cooking time:* 60 minutes

# Baked Sweet Potato Fries

2 sweet potatoes, sliced into
½-inch-thick wedges

1 tablespoon olive oil

½ teaspoon garlic powder

1 teaspoon black pepper

lemon juice, to taste

1. Preheat the oven to 450°F. Grease a baking sheet.

2. In a bowl, combine sweet potato wedges with olive oil and garlic powder until coated. Spread them evenly on the baking sheet.

3. Bake the sweet potato fries for about 15 minutes, and then turn them over and bake another 10 to 15 minutes until they are crispy. If you cut smaller fries, they will take less time to cook.

4. Remove from the oven and sprinkle with black pepper to taste. Gently squeeze lemon juice over the fries to give a light citrus flavor.

*Serves:* 2 to 4

*Prep time:* 10 minutes

*Cooking time:* 30 minutes

# Slow Cooker Spaghetti Squash

1 spaghetti squash, halved

2 cups water

2 tablespoons olive oil

1 teaspoon dried basil

1. Place the spaghetti squash with the water in a slower cooker.

2. Cook on low for 6 to 8 hours. Remove the squash from the heat and let it stand until safe to the touch.

3. Using a spoon or fork, scoop the seeds from the cavity and discard them.

4. Using a fork, shred the inside of the squash like spaghetti strands. Season with olive oil and basil.

*Serves:* 2

*Prep time:* 5 minutes

*Cooking time:* 6 to 8 hours

# Sautéed Swiss Chard

2 tablespoons grapeseed oil

6 cloves garlic, sliced thinly

3 bunches well-rinsed rainbow chard, chopped, ends trimmed

½ teaspoon crushed red pepper flakes

3 tablespoons olive oil

½ lemon, juiced

salt and pepper, to taste

1. In a large pan, heat the grapeseed oil over medium heat.

2. Add the garlic and sauté for 1 minute. Add the chard and season with the red pepper. Cook for 3 minutes, stirring often.

3. Reduce heat to medium low and cover. Cook for 3 more minutes and stir.

4. Cook until chard is tender, 1 or 2 more minutes. Remove from heat. Toss with olive oil and lemon juice. Season with salt and pepper.

*Serves*: 4

*Prep time*: 10 minutes

*Cooking time*: 10 minutes

# Roasted Garlic

1 or more heads garlic                    2 tablespoons olive oil, per head

1. Preheat the oven to 400°F.

2. Peel the outer layer off the garlic as much as possible. Try to keep the head itself intact with the cloves connected.

3. Carefully cut off the very top of the head of garlic, about ¼ inch down, until the tops of the cloves garlic are exposed.

4. Place the garlic in a baking dish lined with parchment paper. Drizzle with the olive oil, letting the oil sink down into the cloves. Wrap over with foil until closed gently and bake for 40 minutes, or until a center clove is soft when pierced with a fork or knife.

*Serves:* 4
*Prep time:* 5 minutes
*Cooking time:* 40 minutes

# Balsamic Dijon Dressing

2 tablespoons olive oil

2 tablespoons balsamic vinegar

1 tablespoons local honey

1 clove garlic, minced

1 teaspoon Dijon mustard

In a small bowl, whisk dressing ingredients. Serve or refrigerate, covered, for up to 2 weeks.

*Serves:* 8
*Prep time:* 3 minutes
*Cooking time:* 0 minutes


# Lemon Vinaigrette

⅓ cup olive oil

¼ cup balsamic vinegar

3 tablespoons lemon juice

4 cloves garlic, minced

½ teaspoon black pepper

In a small bowl, whisk dressing ingredients. Serve or refrigerate, covered, for up to 2 weeks.

*Serves:* 8
*Prep time:* 5 minutes
*Cooking time:* 0 minutes

# DESSERTS

## Easy Fruit Salad

For potassium restriction, use low-potassium fruits such as apples, cranberries, grapes, pineapples, and strawberries.

4 cups chopped pineapple

1 quart halved strawberries

1 cup seedless green grapes

1 cup seedless red grapes

2 mangoes, peeled, cored, and sliced into chunks

4 kiwis, peeled and sliced into chunks

1 pint raspberries

1 pint blueberries

2 tablespoons chopped fresh mint

Wash all of the produce thoroughly and gently pat it dry or allow to drain. Combine in a large bowl and gently mix together. Sprinkle with mint.

*Serves:* 8 to 10

*Prep time:* 20 minutes

*Cooking time:* 0 minutes

# Paleo Brownies

½ cup coconut oil

⅓ cup dark chocolate chips

2 eggs

½ cup maple sugar

½ teaspoon Himalayan sea salt

3 tablespoons arrowroot starch

¼ to ½ cup cacao powder

2 teaspoons vanilla extract

1. Preheat the oven to 350°F.

2. Melt the coconut oil and chocolate chips in a small pot over medium heat.

3. Using a hand mixer, mix all ingredients together until the batter is thick.

4. Pour contents into a 8½ x 4½ x 2¾-inch loaf pan.

5. Bake for 30 minutes.

6. Allow to cool for 15 minutes.

*Serves:* 12

*Prep time:* 10 minutes

*Cooking time:* 30 minutes

# Roasted Pears with Chopped Walnuts

Not ideal for phosphorous restriction.

4 large ripe pears, halved lengthwise, seeds and stems removed

4 teaspoons local honey

½ ground cinnamon

½ cup finely chopped walnuts

1. Preheat the oven to 350°F.

2. Drizzle each pear half with ½ teaspoon of honey and then sprinkle with cinnamon. Top the halves with chopped walnuts.

3. Bake the pears for 30 minutes. Finish under the broiler for 30 seconds to 1 minute for extra crunchy walnuts and a lovely caramelization.

*Serves:* 4

*Prep time:* 5 minutes

*Cooking time:* 30 minutes

# SNACKS

## Bean Dip

1 cup pinto beans

8 ounces full-fat cream cheese

¼ cup olive oil

1 cloves garlic, divided

1 tablespoon ground cumin

¼ teaspoon chili powder

12 ounces sour cream

½ large red onion, finely chopped

1 green bell pepper, finely chopped

1 red bell pepper, finely chopped

2 limes

⅓ cup fresh cilantro

1. Blend the pinto beans, cream cheese, olive oil, 2 cloves garlic, cumin, and chili powder in a food processor or high-speed blender. Spread into a 9 x 9-inch pan.

2. Using a spatula, layer the sour cream over the bean mixture.

3. Lightly sauté the red onion, green and red bell peppers, and remaining garlic clove, minced, in a skillet. Avoid overcooking so that peppers are firm, not mushy.

4. Squeeze limes over sautéed bell peppers and onion mixture for extra flavor. Drain excess liquid.

5. Spoon bell pepper mixture on top of sour cream and smooth over until the dip is covered.

6. Top dish with cilantro.

*Serves:* 8

*Prep time:* 15 minutes

*Cooking time:* 0 minutes

# Deviled Eggs

2 teaspoons canned pimento

2 large hard-boiled eggs, halved, whites and yolks separated

½ teaspoon dry mustard

2 tablespoons avocado mayonnaise

½ teaspoon black pepper

⅛ teaspoon paprika

1. Dice pimento and mix with egg yolk, dry mustard, mayonnaise, and black pepper.

2. Place mixture inside egg white halves in equal parts.

3. Sprinkle eggs with paprika.

*Serves:* 2
*Prep time:* 5 minutes
*Cooking time:* 0 minutes

# Snacky Chickpeas

Not ideal for phosphorous restriction.

1 (15-ounce) can chickpeas, drained and rinsed

½ teaspoon smoked paprika

1 teaspoon olive oil

1. Pat the chickpeas until they are very dry.

2. Preheat the oven to 350°F. Mix all the ingredients together in a bowl, then spread the chickpeas evenly on a baking sheet. Bake in the oven for 45 minutes or until crunchy.

3. Remove from the oven and let cool.

*Serves:* 4
*Prep time:* 5 minutes
*Cooking time:* 45 minutes

# Sweet and Spicy Nuts

Not ideal for phosphorous restriction.

| | |
|---|---|
| cooking spray or grapeseed oil | ⅓ cup maple syrup |
| 3 cups raw cashews | 2 tablespoons brown sugar |
| 2 cups raw walnuts | ½ orange, juiced |
| 2 cups raw pecans | 2 teaspoons chipotle powder |
| ½ cup raw almonds | 2 teaspoons sea salt, divided |

1. Preheat the oven to 350°F. Spray a baking pan with cooking spray or grease the pan lightly with grapeseed oil.

2. In a large bowl, combine the nuts. Add the maple syrup, brown sugar, orange juice, and chipotle powder, and toss well to combine.

3. Spread the nuts in an even layer on the pan. Sprinkle with half of the sea salt.

4. Bake for 25 minutes, or until the nuts are browned, stirring twice. Remove from the oven and sprinkle with the remaining salt. Stir to combine.

5. Let the nuts cool at room temperature, stirring occasionally to prevent sticking. Store in an airtight container.

*Serves:* 10

*Prep time:* 10 minutes

*Cooking time:* 25 minutes

# APPENDIX

## DAILY FOOD LOG

| Date: | | Number of Servings | | | |
|---|---|---|---|---|---|
| Food (include serving size) | Sodium (mg) | Vegetables | Fruits | Grains | Milk/Milk Alternative |
| Breakfast | | | | | |
| Lunch | | | | | |
| Dinner | | | | | |
| Snack 1 | | | | | |
| Snack 2 | | | | | |
| Snack 3 | | | | | |
| Daily Totals | | | | | |
| Recommended daily calories and servings (see chart on page 25) | | | | | |
| Exercise Type: | | | | | |

| Number of Servings | | | | How do you feel? |
|---|---|---|---|---|
| Meats, fish, poultry | Nuts, seeds, legumes | Fats, Oils | Sweets, Added Sugars | |
| | | | | |
| | | | | |
| | | | | |
| | | | | |
| | | | | |
| | | | | |
| | | | | |
| | | | | |
| Duration of Exercise: | | | | |

# Potassium Levels of Selected Foods

## FOODS HIGH IN POTASSIUM (MORE THAN 200 MG)

| Food | Serving | Potassium (mg) |
|------|---------|----------------|
| Apricots | 3 raw or 6 dry | 300 |
| Artichoke, medium | 1 | 345 |
| Avocado | ¼ | 245 |
| Banana, medium | 1 | 425 |
| Beans: lima, baked, canned | ½ cup | 280 |
| Beans, white, canned | ½ cup | 595 |
| Beef, roast | 3 ounces | 320 |
| Beef, ground | 3 ounces | 270 |
| Beets, raw or cooked | ½ cup | 260 |
| Bran muffin | 2 oz | 300 |
| Broccoli | ½ cup | 230 |
| Beans, dried | ½ cup | 300–475 |
| Brussels sprouts | ½ cup | 250 |
| Cantaloupe | ½ cup | 215 |
| Cereal, 100% bran | ½ cup | 200–400 |
| Cheeseburger | 1 | 225–400 |
| Chicken | 3 ounces | 220 |
| Clams, canned | 3 ounces | 535 |
| Crab | 3 ounces | 225 |
| Dates, medium | 5 | 270 |
| Fig, dried | 2 | 260 |
| Fish: halibut, tuna, cod, snapper | 3 ounces | 480 |

## FOODS HIGH IN POTASSIUM (MORE THAN 200 MG)

| Food | Serving | Potassium (mg) |
|------|---------|----------------|
| Fish: salmon, haddock, swordfish, perch | 3 ounces | 300 |
| Fish: tuna, canned | 3 ounces | 200–225 |
| French fries, fast food | 3 ounces/small | 470 |
| Granola with fruit, nuts | ½ cup | 200–250 |
| Grapefruit juice | ½ cup | 200–225 |
| Greens, beet | ½ cup | 655 |
| Honeydew melon | ½ cup | 200–225 |
| Kale, raw | 1 cup | 300 |
| Kiwi, medium | 1 | 240 |
| Kohlrabi | ½ cup | 280 |
| Lentils | ½ cup | 365 |
| Mango | 1 each | 325 |
| Milk, chocolate | 1 cup | 420 |
| Milk: fat free, low fat, whole, buttermilk | 1 cup | 350–380 |
| Molasses | 1 tbsp | 295 |
| Mushrooms | ½ cup | 280 |
| Nectarine | 1 | 275 |
| Nuts: almonds, peanuts, hazelnuts, Brazil, cashew, mixed | 1 ounce | 200–250 |
| Nuts: pistachios | 1 ounce | 295 |
| Orange, medium | 1 | 240 |
| Orange juice | ½ cup | 235 |
| Parsnips | ½ cup | 280 |
| Peas, dried | ½ cup | 300–475 |

## FOODS HIGH IN POTASSIUM (MORE THAN 200 MG)

| Food | Serving | Potassium (mg) |
|------|---------|----------------|
| Papaya, medium | ½ | 390 |
| Peanut butter, chunky | 2 tablespoons | 240 |
| Peanut butter, smooth | 2 tablespoons | 210 |
| Pear, medium | 1 | 200–225 |
| Pomegranate, whole | 1 | 400 |
| Pomegranate juice | ½ cup | 215 |
| Pork | 3 ounces | 350 |
| Potato chips, salted | 1 ounce | 465 |
| Potato, medium, baked with skin | 1 | 925 |
| Potatoes, boiled | ½ cup | 255 |
| Potatoes, mashed | ½ cup | 330 |
| Prune juice | ½ cup | 370 |
| Prunes | 5 | 305 |
| Pudding, chocolate | ½ cup | 230 |
| Pumpkin, canned | ½ cup | 250 |
| Raisins, seedless | ¼ cup | 270 |
| Rutabaga | ½ cup | 280 |
| Seeds: sunflower or pumpkin | 1 ounce | 240 |
| Soy milk | 1 cup | 300 |
| Spinach, canned | ½ cup | 420 |
| Spinach, cooked | ½ cup | 370 |
| Sweet potato, baked with skin, medium | 1 | 450 |
| Swiss chard | ½ cup | 480 |
| Tomato or vegetable juice | ½ cup | 275 |

## FOODS HIGH IN POTASSIUM (MORE THAN 200 MG)

| Food | Serving | Potassium (mg) |
|---|---|---|
| Tomato sauce or puree | ½ cup | 400–550 |
| Tomato, raw, medium | 1 | 290 |
| Tomatoes, canned | ½ cup | 200–300 |
| Turkey | 3 ounces | 250 |
| Wheat germ | 1 ounce | 250 |
| Winter squash | ½ cup | 250 |
| Yogurt: plain or fruited | 6 ounces | 260–435 |
| Zucchini | ½ cup | 220 |

## FOODS MODERATE IN POTASSIUM (50–200 MG)

| Food | Serving | Potassium (mg) |
|---|---|---|
| Apple | 1 each | 150 |
| Apple juice | ½ cup | 150 |
| Applesauce | ½ cup | 90 |
| Apricot nectar | ½ cup | 140 |
| Asparagus | ½ cup or 6 small spears | 155 |
| Bagel, cinnamon raisin | 1 | 130 |
| Bagel: egg or plain | 1 (4") piece | 70 |
| Beans, green | ½ cup | 90 |
| Beans, yellow | ½ cup | 190 |
| Beer, regular | 12 ounces | 100 |
| Beets, canned | ½ cup | 125 |
| Blackberries | ½ cup | 115 |
| Blueberries | ½ cup | 60 |
| Bread, whole wheat | 1 slice | 70 |

## FOODS MODERATE IN POTASSIUM (50–200 MG)

| Food | Serving | Potassium (mg) |
|------|---------|----------------|
| Broccoli, raw | ½ cup | 145 |
| Cabbage | ½ cup | 150 |
| Carrots, cooked or raw | ½ cup | 180 |
| Cauliflower, raw | ½ cup | 150 |
| Celery, raw | ½ cup | 155 |
| Cereal, bran flakes | ½ cup | 120–150 |
| Cheese, cottage | ½ cup | 110 |
| Cherries | 10 | 150 |
| Chocolate | 1½-ounce bar | 165 |
| Coffee, brewed | 6 ounces | 90 |
| Corn | ½ cup or 1 ear | 195 |
| Cucumbers | ½ cup | 80 |
| Egg, large | 1 | 60 |
| Eggplant | ½ cup | 60 |
| Endive, raw | ½ cup | 80 |
| English muffin | 1 | 65 |
| Frankfurter, beef/pork | 1 | 75 |
| Fruit cocktail, canned | ½ cup | 115 |
| Grape juice | ½ cup | 170 |
| Grapefruit | ½ | 175 |
| Grapes | ½ cup | 155 |
| Greens: kale, turnip, collard | ½ cup | 110–150 |
| Ice cream or frozen yogurt, chocolate | ½ cup | 175 |
| Ice cream or frozen yogurt, vanilla | ½ cup | 120–150 |

## FOODS MODERATE IN POTASSIUM (50–200 MG)

| Food | Serving | Potassium (mg) |
|---|---|---|
| Lemon or lime | 1 | 80 |
| Lettuce, all types | 1 cup | 100 |
| Mixed vegetables | ½ cup | 150 |
| Mushrooms, raw | ½ cup | 110 |
| Nuts: walnuts, pecans, macadamia | 1 ounce | 125 |
| Oatmeal | ½ cup | 80 |
| Okra | ½ cup | 110 |
| Onions, raw | ½ cup | 120 |
| Peach | 1 | 185 |
| Peaches, canned | ½ cup | 120 |
| Pears, canned | ½ cup | 120 |
| Peas, green, frozen | ½ cup | 90 |
| Peppers, green | ½ cup | 130 |
| Peppers, red | ½ cup | 160 |
| Pineapple juice | ½ cup | 165 |
| Pineapple, fresh or canned | ½ cup | 100 |
| Plum | 1 | 105 |
| Pudding, vanilla | ½ cup | 150 |
| Raspberries | ½ cup | 90 |
| Rhubarb | ½ cup | 115 |
| Rice, wild | ½ cup | 80 |
| Shrimp | 3 ounces | 155 |
| Spinach, raw | 1 cup | 170 |
| Strawberries | ½ cup | 125 |

## FOODS MODERATE IN POTASSIUM (50–200 MG)

| Food | Serving | Potassium (mg) |
|------|---------|----------------|
| Summer squash | ½ cup | 175–200 |
| Swiss chard, raw | 1 cup | 135 |
| Tangerine | 1 | 140 |
| Tea, brewed | 6 ounces | 65 |
| Turnips | ½ cup | 140 |
| Watermelon | ½ cup | 85 |
| Wine, red, table | 5 ounces | 180 |
| Wine, white, table | 5 ounces | 100 |

## FOODS LOW IN POTASSIUM (LESS THAN 50 MG)

| Food | Serving | Potassium (mg) |
|------|---------|----------------|
| Bread, white | 1 slice | 30 |
| Carbonated beverages | 12 ounces | < 5 |
| Cheese | 1 ounce | 20–30 |
| Cranberries | ½ cup | 45 |
| Cranberry juice cocktail | ½ cup | 20 |
| Fats and oils | 1 tbsp | < 5 |
| Hummus | 1 tbsp | 32 |
| Nectar, papaya, mango, or pear | ½ cup | 35 |
| Rice, white or brown | ½ cup | 40–50 |
| Spaghetti/macaroni, cooked | ½ cup | 30 |
| Tortilla, flour or corn | 1 | 40–50 |
| Waffle | 1 (4") | 40–50 |
| Water chestnuts | ½ cup | 40 |

Source: © 2018 Academy of Nutrition and Dietetics, Nutrition Care Manual®. Accessed July 10, 2017. Adapted and reprinted with permission.

# Phosphorus Levels of Selected Foods

## HIGH PHOSPHORUS FOODS (MORE THAN 100 MG)

| Food | Serving | mg |
|------|---------|-----|
| Almonds | 1 oz | 140 |
| Biscuit | 4" piece | 140 |
| Beans and peas, cooked or canned | ½ cup | 100–140 |
| Beef or veal | 3 ounces | 200 |
| Cereal, bran | ½ cup | 140–350 |
| Cheese: American, cheddar, mozzarella, Swiss, provolone | 1 ounce | 150 |
| Chicken, white meat | 3 ounces | 200 |
| Milk, condensed, sweetened | ½ cup | 390 |
| Cheese, ricotta | ½ cup | 225 |
| Cheese, cottage | ½ cup | 170 |
| Cream, light or half-and-half | ½ cup | 110 |
| Milk, evaporated | ½ cup | 260 |
| Fish: pollock, walleye, swordfish, cod, halibut, salmon, tuna | 3 ounces | 200–280 |
| Granola | ½ cup | 150 |
| Hot cocoa, prepared | 6 ounces | 100–150 |
| Lentils | ½ cup | 180 |
| Milk, all kinds | 1 cup | 240 |
| Milkshake | 1 cup | 260 |
| Nuts, most varieties | 1 ounce | 100–130 |
| Oatmeal | ½ cup | 160 |

## HIGH PHOSPHORUS FOODS (MORE THAN 100 MG)

| Food | Serving | mg |
|---|---|---|
| Organ meats | 1 oz | 125 |
| Oysters, medium | 3 | 180 |
| Peanut/nut butters | 2 tablespoons | 115 |
| Pork, loin | 3 oz | 200 |
| Potato, medium, baked with skin | 1 | 120 |
| Pudding or custard, made with milk | ½ cup | 150 |
| Sardines | 3 ounces | 420 |
| Seeds, sunflower or pumpkin | 1 ounce | 340 |
| Shrimp or crab | 3 ounces | 110 |
| Soybeans | ½ cup | 210 |
| Soy milk | 1 cup | 130 |
| Tofu, firm | ¼ block | 100–150 |
| Tortilla, corn | 2 (6") pieces | 120 |
| Tuna, canned in water, drained | 3 ounces | 140 |
| Turkey, light or dark | 3 ounces | 180 |
| Veggie or soy patty | 1 patty | 145 |
| Wheat germ | 1 tablespoon | 115 |
| Waffle or pancake | 4" piece | 120 |
| Yogurt, plain or with fruit | 6 ounces | 220–360 |

## MODERATE PHOSPHORUS (50–100 MG)

| Food | Serving | mg |
|---|---|---|
| Asparagus | ½ cup | 45 |
| Bacon | 2 slices | 70 |
| Bagel | 1 (3") piece | 50 |

## MODERATE PHOSPHORUS (50–100 MG)

| Food | Serving | mg |
|---|---|---|
| Beans, baked | ½ cup | 95 |
| Beer or ale | 12 ounces | 50 |
| Bread, whole wheat | 1 slice | 55 |
| Cake | 2×2" piece | 90 |
| Cereal, non-bran | ½ cup | 50–100 |
| Cheese, Parmesan | 2 tablespoons | 90 |
| Chocolate | 1.5-ounce bar | 90 |
| Cocoa | 2 tablespoons | 80 |
| Cookies, sandwich type | 4 | 40 |
| Corn | ½ cup | 65 |
| Egg, large | 1 | 95 |
| English muffin | 1 | 50 |
| Granola bar, hard, plain | 1 bar | 70 |
| Ice milk, ice cream, or frozen yogurt | ½ cup | 75 |
| Iced tea, canned | 12 ounces | 95 |
| Muffin | 2 ounces | 75 |
| Mushrooms | ½ cup | 60 |
| Pasta or noodles, egg | ½ cup | 60 |
| Peas, green | ½ cup | 65 |
| Rice, brown or wild | ½ cup | 75 |
| Salami | 1 ounce | 65 |
| Spaghetti, whole wheat | ½ cup | 65 |
| Spinach | ½ cup | 50 |
| Sweet potato, medium, baked with skin | 1 | 60 |

## LOW PHOSPHORUS (LESS THAN 50 MG)

| Food | Serving | mg |
|---|---|---|
| Beans, green or yellow | ½ cup | 20 |
| Bread, pumpernickel or rye | 1 slice | 45 |
| Bread, white | 1 slice | 25 |
| Brussels sprouts | ½ cup | 45 |
| Candy, hard or jelly beans | 1 ounce | 5 |
| Caramels | 1 ounce | 30 |
| Cereals: rice and corn | 1 cup | 20 |
| Cheese, cream | 1 ounce | 30 |
| Coffee, brewed | 6 ounces | 5 |
| Cream of wheat or grits | ½ cup | 20 |
| Creamer, nondairy, liquid | 1 ounce | 20 |
| Fats and oils | 1 tablespoon | < 5 |
| Fruit juices | ½ cup | 15–30 |
| Fruit, most types | 1 piece or ½ cup | < 30 |
| Gelatin | ½ cup | 30 |
| Greens | ½ cup | 30 |
| Malt, chocolate mix | 1 tablespoon | 35 |
| Popcorn, air popped | 1 cup | 30 |
| Popsicles or juice bars | 1 bar | 0 |
| Pretzels | 1 ounce | 30 |
| Pudding or custard, ready to eat | ½ cup | 45 |
| Rice, white | ½ cup | 35 |
| Sausage, pork | 1 ounce | 40 |
| Sherbet | ½ cup | 30 |

## LOW PHOSPHORUS (LESS THAN 50 MG)

| Food | Serving | mg |
|------|---------|-----|
| Soda: cola or dark-type | 12 ounces | 40–50 |
| Soda: lemon-lime, ginger ale | 12 ounces | 0 |
| Spaghetti or macaroni | ½ cup | 40 |
| Spaghetti squash | ½ cup | 11 |
| Spinach | ½ cup | 40–50 |
| Tea, black, brewed | 6 ounces | 2 |
| Tomato, raw | 1 medium | 30 |
| Wine, all varieties | 5 ounces | 30 |

Source: © 2018 Academy of Nutrition and Dietetics, Nutrition Care Manual®. Accessed July 10, 2017. Adapted and reprinted with permission.

# Sample Meal Plans

## 3-DAY DASH MEAL PLAN EXAMPLE

|  | Breakfast | Lunch | Dinner | Snack |
|---|---|---|---|---|
| **Day 1** | Veggie Omelet *(page 115)* with ½ avocado | Spicy Baked Fish *(page 125)* with ¼ cup brown rice | Spinach Salad *(page 127)* | Sweet and Spicy Nuts *(page 164)* |
| **Day 2** | Nutty Overnight Oats *(page 118)* | Pasta Primavera *(page 136)* | Lemon Rosemary Chicken Skillet *(page 130)* | Snacky Chickpeas *(page 163)* |
| **Day 3** | Greek Yogurt Parfait *(page 120)* | Couscous and Veggies *(page 129)* | Grilled Chicken Paillard *(page 132)* | Deviled Eggs *(page 163)* |

## 3-DAY CKD MEAL PLAN EXAMPLE

|  | Breakfast | Lunch | Dinner | Snack |
|---|---|---|---|---|
| **Day 1** | Banana Oat Shake *(page 113)* | Lemony Vegetable and Rice Salad *(page 122)* | Couscous and Veggies *(page 129)* | Peaches with whipped cream: ½ cup unsweetened canned peaches with 2 tablespoons nondairy whipped topping |
| **Day 2** | Veggie Omelet *(page 115)* | Fiesta Lime Ground Turkey *(page 123)* | Pasta Primavera *(page 136)* | Chilled or frozen grapes |
| **Day 3** | Berry Overnight Oats *(page 117)* | Spicy Baked Fish *(page 125)* | Vegetable Green Curry *(page 141)* | Lemon cookies |

# 3-DAY DIALYSIS MEAL PLAN EXAMPLE

|  | Breakfast | Lunch | Dinner | Snack |
|---|---|---|---|---|
| Day 1 | Cranberry juice, 4 oz. 2 eggs with 2 slices toasted white bread with butter | Tuna salad sandwich on a hard roll with lettuce and mayonnaise Low-salt pretzels Ginger ale, 8 oz. | Hamburger on a bun with 1–2 teaspoons ketchup | Sliced apples |
| Day 2 | Breakfast burrito with 2 eggs, onion, broccoli, and peppers rolled up in a 6-inch white tortilla | Chicken salad on white bread Carrot sticks | Large salad with lettuce, cucumbers, radishes, and peppers with olive oil and apple cider vinegar dressing | Low-sodium crackers |
| Day 3 | Cranberry juice, 4 oz. Toasted bagel with 2 tablespoons cream cheese | Canned salmon salad | 3 oz. roasted chicken ½ cup white rice 1 cooked cup carrots and peas | Fresh pineapple |

# Meal Planning Chart

| Breakfast | Protein | Phosphorous | Potassium | Sodium | Fluid |
|---|---|---|---|---|---|
|  |  |  |  |  |  |
|  |  |  |  |  |  |
|  |  |  |  |  |  |
| Lunch |  |  |  |  |  |
|  |  |  |  |  |  |
|  |  |  |  |  |  |
|  |  |  |  |  |  |
| Dinner |  |  |  |  |  |
|  |  |  |  |  |  |
|  |  |  |  |  |  |
|  |  |  |  |  |  |

DASH Diet *for* Renal Health

| Snack | | | | | |
|---|---|---|---|---|---|
| | | | | | |
| | | | | | |
| | | | | | |
| Total | | | | | |
| Recommended | _____ g | _____ mg | _____ mg | _____ mg | _____ oz |

# Food Shopping List

Write in the quantity/volume needed on the blank line.

**VEGETABLES** (Fresh or frozen preferred to canned; if canned, drain and rinse well)

- ❏ _____ Alfalfa sprouts
- ❏ _____ Artichoke
- ❏ _____ Arugula
- ❏ _____ Asparagus
- ❏ _____ Avocados
- ❏ _____ Beets
- ❏ _____ Bell peppers
- ❏ _____ Bok choy
- ❏ _____ Broccoli
- ❏ _____ Broccoli rabe
- ❏ _____ Brussels sprouts
- ❏ _____ Cabbage
- ❏ _____ Carrots
- ❏ _____ Cauliflower
- ❏ _____ Celery
- ❏ _____ Collard greens
- ❏ _____ Cucumbers
- ❏ _____ Eggplant
- ❏ _____ Endive lettuce
- ❏ _____ Garlic
- ❏ _____ Green beans

☐ _____ Jerusalem artichoke

☐ _____ Kale

☐ _____ Mushrooms

☐ _____ Okra

☐ _____ Olives

☐ _____ Onions

☐ _____ Parsnips

☐ _____ Peppers

☐ _____ Pumpkin

☐ _____ Purple potatoes

☐ _____ Radish

☐ _____ Red potatoes

☐ _____ Romaine lettuce

☐ _____ Sea vegetables

☐ _____ Scallions

☐ _____ Spinach

☐ _____ Squash

☐ _____ Sweet potatoes

☐ _____ Tomatoes

☐ _____ Watercress

☐ _____ Wheat grass

## FRUITS

☐ _____ Apple

☐ _____ Apricot

☐ _____ Banana

❑ _____ Blackberries

❑ _____ Blueberries

❑ _____ Cantaloupe

❑ _____ Cherries

❑ _____ Coconuts

❑ _____ Cranberries

❑ _____ Figs

❑ _____ Goji berries

❑ _____ Grapefruit

❑ _____ Grapes

❑ _____ Lemon

❑ _____ Lime

❑ _____ Mango

❑ _____ Nectarine

❑ _____ Orange

❑ _____ Papaya

❑ _____ Peaches

❑ _____ Pears

❑ _____ Pineapple

❑ _____ Plums

❑ _____ Pomegranate

❑ _____ Raspberries

❑ _____ Rhubarb

❑ _____ Strawberries

❑ _____ Watermelon

## SEAFOOD

- ❑ _____ Anchovies
- ❑ _____ Bass
- ❑ _____ Cod
- ❑ _____ Grouper
- ❑ _____ Halibut
- ❑ _____ Herring
- ❑ _____ Mackerel
- ❑ _____ Mahi mahi
- ❑ _____ Red snapper
- ❑ _____ Salmon (canned or fresh)
- ❑ _____ Sardines
- ❑ _____ Shrimp
- ❑ _____ Tuna (packed in water)

## DAIRY/DAIRY ALTERNATIVES

- ❑ _____ Organic cow's milk
- ❑ _____ Goat's milk
- ❑ _____ Kefir
- ❑ _____ Unsweetened coconut milk
- ❑ _____ Unsweetened cashew milk
- ❑ _____ Unsweetened almond milk

## MEAT/MEAT ALTERNATIVES

- ❑ _____ Beef
- ❑ _____ Bison
- ❑ _____ Chicken

- ❑ _____ Duck
- ❑ _____ Eggs
- ❑ _____ Lamb
- ❑ _____ Tempeh
- ❑ _____ Turkey
- ❑ _____ Turkey bacon

## NUTS AND SEEDS

- ❑ _____ Almonds
- ❑ _____ Brazil nuts
- ❑ _____ Chia seeds
- ❑ _____ Flaxseeds
- ❑ _____ Hemp seeds
- ❑ _____ Hazelnuts
- ❑ _____ Macadamia nuts
- ❑ _____ Pecans
- ❑ _____ Pine nuts
- ❑ _____ Pistachios
- ❑ _____ Pumpkin seeds
- ❑ _____ Sesame seeds
- ❑ _____ Walnuts
- ❑ _____ Nut butters
- ❑ _____ Seed butters

## FATS/OILS

- ❑ _____ Avocado oil
- ❑ _____ Almond oil
- ❑ _____ Butter (grass-fed)
- ❑ _____ Coconut oil
- ❑ _____ Ghee
- ❑ _____ Grapeseed oil
- ❑ _____ Olive oil
- ❑ _____ Sesame oil
- ❑ _____ Walnut oil

## GRAINS/STARCHES

- ❑ _____ Amaranth
- ❑ _____ Barley
- ❑ _____ Brown rice
- ❑ _____ Brown rice pasta
- ❑ _____ Einkorn pasta
- ❑ _____ Beans (all kinds)
- ❑ _____ Chickpea pasta
- ❑ _____ Lentil pasta
- ❑ _____ Flax bread
- ❑ _____ Farro
- ❑ _____ Lentils
- ❑ _____ Muesli

❑ _____ Oats

❑ _____ Spelt

❑ _____ Sprouted grain tortillas

❑ _____ Teff

❑ _____ Quinoa

❑ _____ Wild rice

## SPICES AND HERBS

❑ _____ Basil

❑ _____ Black pepper

❑ _____ Cayenne pepper

❑ _____ Chili pepper

❑ _____ Cilantro

❑ _____ Coriander seeds

❑ _____ Cinnamon

❑ _____ Cloves

❑ _____ Cumin

❑ _____ Dill

❑ _____ Fennel

❑ _____ Garlic

❑ _____ Ginger

❑ _____ Mint

❑ _____ Mustard seeds

❑ _____ Nutmeg

❑ _____ Oregano

❑ _____ Paprika

- ❑ _____ Parsley
- ❑ _____ Peppermint
- ❑ _____ Rosemary
- ❑ _____ Sage
- ❑ _____ Tarragon
- ❑ _____ Thyme
- ❑ _____ Turmeric
- ❑ _____ Mrs. Dash seasoning
- ❑ _____ Seasoning blends (low-sodium or salt-free without added potassium)

## CONDIMENTS

- ❑ _____ Apple cider vinegar
- ❑ _____ Balsamic vinegar
- ❑ _____ Coconut amino acids
- ❑ _____ Extracts (vanilla/almond)
- ❑ _____ Guacamole
- ❑ _____ Hummus
- ❑ _____ Mustard
- ❑ _____ Mayo (avocado oil)
- ❑ _____ Salsa
- ❑ _____ Pink Himalayan salt
- ❑ _____ Tamari
- ❑ _____ Raw honey
- ❑ _____ Stevia

# REFERENCES

Academy of Nutrition and Dietetics. Nutrition Care Manual. http://www.nutritioncaremanual.org. Accessed July 10, 2017.

Borghi, Loris, Tania Schianchi, et al. "Comparison of Two Diets for the Prevention of Recurrent Stones in Idiopathic Hypercalciuria." *New England Journal of Medicine* 346, no. 2 (2002): 77-84. doi:10.1056.

Center for Food Safety and Applied Nutrition. "Labeling & Nutrition: Changes to the Nutrition Facts Label." United States Food and Drug Administration. https://www.fda.gov/Food/GuidanceRegulation/GuidanceDocumentsRegulatoryInformation/LabelingNutrition/ucm385663.htm. Retrieved July 4, 2017.

Center for Mindful Eating. "The Principles of Mindful Eating." https://www.thecenterformindfuleating.org/Principles-Mindful-Eating. Retrieved May 4, 2017.

Chiu, Sally, Nathalie Bergeron, et al. "Comparison of the Dash (Dietary Approaches to Stop Hypertension) Diet and a Higher-Fat Dash Diet on Blood Pressure and Lipids and Lipoproteins: a Randomized Controlled Trial." *American Journal of Clinical Nutrition*, Volume 103, Issue 2 (2016): 341–347. doi:10.3945/ajcn.115.123281.

Cleveland Clinic. "Kidney Stones: Oxalate-Controlled Diet." February 17, 2015. https://my.clevelandclinic.org/health/articles/kidney-stones-oxalate-controlled-diet. Retrieved June 9, 2017.

Colman, Sara. "Best Cereal Choices for the Kidney Diet." DaVita.com. July 9, 2010. http://blogs.davita.com/kidney-diet-tips/best-cereal-choices-for-the-kidney-diet. Retrieved July 3, 2017.

DaVita Kidney Care. "Dietary Protein and Chronic Kidney Disease." DaVita.com. https://www.davita.com/kidney-disease/diet-and-nutrition/ diet-basics/dietary-protein-and-chronic-kidney-disease/e/5302. Retrieved May 12, 2017.

DaVita Kidney Care. "Potassium and Chronic Kidney Disease." DaVita .com. https://www.davita.com/kidney-disease/diet-and-nutrition/ diet%20basics/potassium-and-chronic-kidney-disease/e/5308. Retrieved September 10, 2017.

Erdman Jr., John W., LeaAnn Carson, et al. "Effects of Cocoa Flavanols on Risk Factors for Cardiovascular Disease." *Asia Pacific Journal of Clinical Nutrition*, 17 (2008): 284S–287. https://www.ncbi.nlm.nih .gov/pubmed/18296357.

Group, Edward. "What Are Phytochemicals? Discovering Their Health Benefits." Global Healing Center. November 3, 2016. https://www.globalhealingcenter.com/natural-health/what-are- phytochemicals/#1. Retrieved June 10, 2017.

Harris, Cheryl. "Mindful Eating; Studies Show This Concept Can Help Clients Lose Weight and Better Manage Chronic Disease." *Today's Dietician*, Volume 15, Issue 3 (March 2013). http://www. todaysdietitian.com/newarchives/030413p42.shtml.

Harvard Heart Letter. "Potassium and Sodium Out of Balance." Harvard Health Publishing. April 2009. https://www.health.harvard.edu/ newsletter_article/Potassium_and_sodium_out_of_balance. Retrieved December 4, 2017.

Hyman, Mark. "Good Fats vs. Bad Fats: Dr. Hyman's Healthy Cheat Sheet." *The Chalkboard*. March 11, 2016. http://thechalkboardmag. com/dr-hyman-good-fat-bad-fat. Retrieved July 10, 2017.

Jakobsen, Marianne U., Claus Dethlefsen, et al. "Intake of Carbohydrates Compared with Intake of Saturated Fatty Acids and Risk of Myocardial Infarction: Importance of the Glycemic Index." *American Journal of Clinical Nutrition*, Volume 91, Issue 6 (June 2010): 1764–8. doi: 10.3945/ajcn.2009.29099.

Kibangou, Ida B., Saïd Bouhallab, et al. "Milk Proteins and Iron Absorption: Contrasting Effects of Different Caseinophosphopeptides." *Pediatric Research*, Volume 58, Issue 4 (2005): 731–4. doi: 10.1203/01.PDR.0000180555.27710.46.

Krewski, Daniel, Robert A. Yokel, et al. "Human Health Risk Assessment for Aluminium, Aluminium Oxide, and Aluminium Hydroxide." *Journal of Toxicology & Environmental Health: Part B*, Volume 10, Issue 1 (2007): 101. doi:10.1080/10937400701597766.

Krinsky, Norman I., John T. Landrum, et al. "Biologic Mechanisms of the Protective Role of Lutein and Zeaxanthin in the Eye." *Annual Review of Nutrition*, Volume 23, Issue 1 (2003): 171–201. doi: 10.1146/annurev.nutr.23.011702.073307.

Lewis, James L. "Overview of Electrolytes." Merck. https://www.merck manuals.com/home/hormonal-and-metabolic-disorders/electrolyte-balance/overview-of-electrolytes. Retrieved July 4, 2017.

Mahan, L. Kathleen, Janice L. Raymond, et al. *Krause's Food and the Nutrition Care Process*. New York: Elsevier Health Sciences, 2013.

Martin, William, Lawrence Armstrong, et al. "Dietary Protein Intake and Renal Function." *Nutrition & Metabolism*, Volume 2, Issue 25 (September 20, 2005): 2-25. doi: 10.1186/1743-7075-2-25.

May, Michelle. *Eat What You Love, Love What You Eat*. Austin, TX: Greenleaf Book Group Press, 2013.

Mercola, Joseph. *Fat for Fuel: A Revolutionary Diet to Combat Cancer, Boost Brain Power, and Increase Your Energy*. Carlsbad, CA: Hay House, 2017.

Mercola, Joseph. "How to Prevent and Treat Kidney Health with Food," Mercola.com. February 15, 2016. http://articles.mercola.com/sites/articles/archive/2016/02/15/foods-for-kidney-health.aspx. Retrieved July 4, 2017.

Miller, Carla K., Jean L. Kristeller, et al. "Comparative Effectiveness of a Mindful Eating Intervention to a Diabetes Self-Management Intervention among Adults with Type 2 Diabetes: A Pilot Study." *Journal of the Academy of Nutrition and Dietetics*, Volume 112, Issue 11 (2012): 1835–1842. doi:10.1016/j.jand.2012.07.036.

Moreno Franco, B., M. León Latre, et al. "Soluble and Insoluble Dietary Fibre Intake and Risk Factors for Metabolic Syndrome and Cardiovascular Disease in Middle-Aged Adults: the AWHS." *Nutrición Hospitalaria*, Volume 30, Issue 6 (2014): 1279–88. doi:10.3305/ nh.2014.30.6.7778.

National Heart, Lung, and Blood Institute. "DASH Eating Plan." US Department of Health and Human Services. Accessed January 12, 2018. https://www.nhlbi.nih.gov/health-topics/dash-eating-plan.

National Heart, Lung, and Blood Institute. "In Brief: Your Guide to Lowering Your Blood Pressure with DASH." Revised August, 2015. https://www.nhlbi.nih.gov/files/docs/public/heart/dash_brief.pdf.

National Institute of Diabetes and Digestive and Kidney Diseases. "Anemia in Chronic Kidney Disease." National Institutes of Health. July 1, 2014. https://www.niddk.nih.gov/health-information/kidney-disease/ chronic-kidney-disease-ckd/anemia. Retrieved June 20, 2017.

National Institutes of Health. "Sodium/Potassium Ratio Linked to Cardio-vascular Disease Risk." March 18, 2016. https://www.nih.gov/ news-events/nih-research-matters/sodium/potassium-ratio-linked-cardiovascular-disease-risk. Retrieved July 5, 2017.

National Kidney Foundation. "Diabetes; A Major Risk for Kidney Disease." https://www.kidney.org/atoz/content/diabetes.

National Kidney Foundation. "Understanding Your Lab Values." https:// www.kidney.org/atoz/content/understanding-your-lab-values.

National Kidney Foundation. "Your Guide to the New Food Label." February, 3, 2017. https://www.kidney.org/atoz/content/foodlabel. Retrieved June 4, 2017.

Pandey, Kanti Bhooshan and Syed Ibrahim Rizvi. "Plant Polyphenols as Dietary Antioxidants in Human Health and Disease." *Oxidative*

*Medicine and Cellular Longevity,* Volume 2, Issue 5 (2009): 270–78. doi:10.4161/oxim.2.5.9498.

Renal & Urology News. "DASH-style Diet Effective in Preventing, Delaying CKD Progression." http://www.renalandurologynews.com/ nutrition/dash-style-diet-effective-in-preventing-delaying-ckd-progression/ article/243706. Retrieved August 11, 2017.

Stauffer, Melissa E. and Tao Fan. "Prevalence of Anemia in Chronic Kidney Disease in the United States." *PLoS One.* January 2, 2014, doi:https://doi.org/10.1371/journal.pone.0084943.

Taylor, Erin, Teresa T. Fung, et al. "DASH-style Diet Associates with Reduced Risk for Kidney Stones." *Journal of the American Society of Nephrology,* Volume 20, Issue 10 (2009): 2253–2259. doi:10.1681/ ASN.2009030276.

Tobian, L. "Dietary Sodium Chloride and Potassium Have Effects on the Pathophysiology of Hypertension in Humans and Animals." *American Journal of Clinical Nutrition,* Volume 2, (1997): 606S-611S. https:// www.ncbi.nlm.nih.gov/pubmed/9022555.

Williams, Caroline, Claudio Ronco, et al. "Whole Grains in the Renal Diet; Is It Time to Reevaluate Their Role?" *Blood Purification,* Volume 36, Issue 3–4 (2014): 210–214, doi:10.1159/000356683.

Xiao, Chao Wu. "Health Effects of Soy Protein and Isoflavones in Humans." *Journal of Nutrition,* Volume 138, Issue 6 (2008): 1244S-9S. https://www.ncbi.nlm.nih.gov/pubmed/18492864.

# INDEX

sauces, 150–58; snacks, 162–64

Red wine, 70. *See also* Alcohol

Renin, 6, 7

Renin-angiotensin-aldosterone hormonal system, 6–7

Resveratrol, 70

Roasted Cauliflower, 152

Roasted Garlic, 157

Roasted Pears with Chopped Walnuts, 161

SAD. *See* Standard American Diet

Salt in diet, 33–41; chemical composition, 34; natural, 33–34; and potassium balance, 36; suggested restrictions, 39–41; and water balance, 33

Salt substitutes, 40

"Salty six" foods, 38–39

Sandwiches, and sodium levels, 38–39

Sauce recipes, 150–58

Sautéed Swiss Chard, 156

Seafood, 67; recommended daily serving, 24, 25

Secondary hyperparathyroidism, 47

Seeds, 67; recommended daily serving, 24, 26

Serum albumin test, and kidney health, 12

Serum creatinine test, and kidney health, 12

Serving size. *See* Portion size

Shopping, 106–109; list, 184–91; online, 107; recommended brands, 109

Short daily hemodialysis (SDHD), 76

Side dish recipes, 150–58

Slow Cooker Chicken and White Bean Chili, 124

Slow Cooker Spaghetti Squash, 155

SMART goals, 85–87

Snacks, 84; recipes, 162–64

Snacky Chickpeas, 163

Sodium and sodium levels, 6, 7, 54–56: and blood pressure, 17–18; and dialysis, 78; and dining out, 102–104; and evolution, 34–35; industry terms, 101–102; and kidneys, 7, 36–37; and Nutrition Facts label, 100; restrictions, 5, 38–41; and SAD, 35–36; supermarket tips, 108 109, 110. *See also* High-sodium alternatives

Sodium chloride. *See* Salt in diet; Sodium

Soluble fiber, 96, 97

Soups, canned, and sodium levels, 39

Soy products (isoflavones), 70

# ACKNOWLEDGMENTS

First and foremost, this book is dedicated to my Mama, for igniting the fire to my passion for nutrition; for showing me that good health and wellness can heal any ailment.

To Daddy, an avid reader who inspires me to never stop learning.

To Gina and Louie, for the endless support and love.

To Enzo, for being my backbone from the very start of my career; for being right by my side as we go through this journey of life, love, and business together.

To Luna, for keeping my lap warm and giving me puppy kisses through the entire book process.

This is for you all, my family, who I love with my entire heart and strive to make you proud.

And, to Rose, my mentor, who has lead me to follow the less traditional and holistic path of nutrition and dietetics; who has shared her incredible knowledge with me and always encouraged me to follow my heart.

—Sara

# ABOUT THE AUTHORS

**Sara Monk Rivera** is a Registered Dietitian who has dedicated her life to spreading awareness of real food nutrition to help people find freedom from chronic health conditions and harmful dieting. Sara is the founder of her private practice, Mindful Meals Nutrition Services, LLC, where she provides her patients with nutritional counseling and education. To learn more, please visit: www.dietitiansara.com.

**Kristin Diversi**, author of *The MIND Diet Cookbook*, is a writer, editor, and nutritionist. She became interested in health and wellness after seeing the role they played in the well-being of the people she loved, sparking a lifelong dedication to learning more about the subjects. She achieved her Master of Science in Nutrition and Food Sciences from Montclair State University in 2013, with a focus on working with children who were neophobic—or picky eaters. Kristin has worked in the public sector, teaching nutrition education, and as a private nutrition consultant. She is featured regularly in health and wellness publications and believes that wellness is a whole-body effort that everyone can achieve.